Bowel Nosode Materia Medica

2nd edition

Contents:

Bacillus No 7

The keynote symptom of this remedy is extreme weakness or fatigue.

In this remedy, we have extreme mental and physical weakness often out of proportion to the apparent cause and we homoeopaths see more of this in our clinics in these stressful times. The patient seems to overreact to emotional or intellectual pressure but rather than output more energy to deal with the pressure, or being unable to do so, they withdraw into themselves into a state we usually associate with the most severe acids or even into an Opium-type withdrawal from life and its cares. They may also become rigidly fixed in their ideas and behaviours as part of their overreaction.

The symptoms we see may include the obvious physical ones where standing may tire them out and exertion makes them faint but they may also show these symptoms more insidiously as well where movement becomes sluggish without them realizing it. They tend to get steadily slower in their occupation and when they finally stop they just can do no more. They can mow the lawn, but have no energy left to put the mower away afterwards.

Overall patients and their loved ones may report a slow onset weakness and a tendency to reduce activity leading to debility and eventually showing in a wasting of muscle groups.

This weakness may come on after a serious illness or as a result of overindulgence in social drugs including alcohol, especially port, sherry and dark rum.

As a corollary to this weakness and if it is allowed to persist the patient may enter a state similar to Alzheimer's disease with the mental faculties being variable in their acuity depending on the underlying energy of the patient. They may also suffer from fugue states where they become unaware of their surroundings.

In less obvious presentations of the symptoms the patient may merely seem unusually tense and tired. They become too tired to go places and do things they would normally have found pleasure in. They show or experience no enjoyment. This also applies to intimate relations and they may betray little in the way of emotions because they lack the energy to express them. They also may become apathetic and cease complaining about problems or troubles. This patient often presents with few definite symptoms and finding repertorisable symptoms is difficult. In more serious cases the patient may respond dully and without apparent expectation of improvement. They are, and remain, gloomy.

When they are just about coping in the world you will still notice that everything works too slowly even answering your questions seems to wear him out. Their partner may report that they may fall asleep whilst conversing, let alone during sex or they may drift off whilst thinking of an answer to the questions you ask in the consultation. He may also forget what he has just said or what you had asked. Other authors have suggested they suffer ailments after debauchery or sexual activity but my experience is that they are rarely capable of such activity to any great degree and in any case their body is too weak even if the spirit were willing.

Therapeutically you may use this remedy in cases of fatigue, or M.E.

It is indicated in many cases of Alzheimer's disease and premature senility.

Thyrotoxicosis, Gout when accompanied by debility, Asthma with prostration and Osteoporosis from lack of exertion. Spondylitis, rheumatoid and osteoarthritis. It is also useful in children and young people when tonsillitis leaves them with great prostration and lassitude and a slow recovery.

Generalities

Fatigue and physical exhaustion

Muscles stiffen and both muscles and joints crack on movement and are weak. Joints and muscles are worse in the chill and damp and are sensitive to draughts and the patient himself is worse for chill and draught. Their body functions seize up, and seem older than their age would lead you to expect. Complaints often begin, or are worse, in the middle of the night.

Syncope	low blood pressure
Slow pulse	slow to recover
Emaciation	bad reactions to stimulants

The patient may sweat excessively as a concomitant to any complaints and this is worse in humid conditions.

Head

Vertigo after exertion or long standing.

Dull headaches

Scalp may be cracked and dry with brittle hair

Eyes

Tendency to close eyes either because of perpetual tiredness or from oedema of the lids.

Thrombosis of retina

Ears

Catarrhal deafness

Nose

Catarrh but no significant identifiers.

Face

Dusky and puffy, or pallid.

Throat

Tonsillitis with copious mucous.

Chest and Heart

Myocardial insufficiency- arrest from muscle weakness

Slow pulse, low blood pressure.

Cardiac oedema.

Back and neck

Rheumatic pains. General backache better for warmth. Arthritic pain worse for movement. Torticollis. Cracking noises on movement. Worse in cold and damp situations or weather.

Respiration and lungs

Sticky, thick and adhesive mucous that is difficult to raise.

Bronchitis. Asthma. Breathing worse at 2 am

Abdomen

Ptosis of abdomen. Incarcerated flatus.

Flatulent distension after food. Noisy rumblings

Better for eructations.

Tenderness or pain in area of liver

Stomach and digestion

Aversion to meat fat.

Borborygmus with copious and loud eructations of air.

Slow to eat, slower to digest food.

Female

Metrorrhagia and menorrhagia.

Conception difficult.

Copious leucorrhoea.

Male

Poor erectile function

Copious ejaculation.

Rectum and Stool

Constipation. Slow to pass stool. Difficult stool even when soft. Haemorrhoids

Anal prolapse. Interstitial prolapse

Kidneys and Urinary

Slow flow of urine

Sleep and dreams

It may take them two hours to go off into a light sleep and they may wake between 2-3am. In general, they are worse around 2am if they have been unable to sleep but I have also noted weariness at 2pm in several patients.

Extremities

Swollen limbs especially lower limbs. Left sided gout.
Rheumatic pains and cramps in wrists and lower limbs.
Shooting nerve pains in legs
Paralysis of wrists and ankles. Noisy joints.
Cracked palms.
Varicose veins large but usually painless.
Dropped arches.

Skin

Circinate eruptions on the palms.
Cracked fingertips and knuckles.
Scaly eruptions on palms.
Sensitive skin.

General Modalities

< after eating
< even thinking about exertion, beginning exertion.
< damp, cold
> heat and rest

Related remedies

Arsenicum album	Bromium	Calcarea Carbonica
Calcarea fluorica	Causticum	Iodine
Kali Carbonicum	Kali Iodatum	Rhus Toxicodendron

Bacillus no 10

The keynote use of Bacillus 10 is ailments from internal trauma including poisoning
Almost any complaints which produce derangement of the system from severe mental trauma or physical damage to the digestive or eliminative organs can be improved by Bacillus 10.

The basic character of these patients is anxious and self-critical, with a tendency to be easily depressed. They are obsessive and fastidious. These characteristics may be aggravated by trauma or may be new symptoms indicating the need for the remedy. When sick all their mental and physical processes seem to become sluggish and their whole personality becomes heavy.

There tend to be a broad variety of symptoms and I have used it to get cases moving or even completely cure patients after inhalation of poison gas, as in Gulf War syndrome, or simply inhalation of poisonous weed killer fumes in gardeners I have also used it successfully in patients with severe headaches after inhalation of paint fumes or headaches and debility from use of toxic cleaning fluids as in engine cleaners for vehicles or aircraft.

In my local farming community, I have used it where there has been a causation of inhalation of sheep dip chemicals which produced overall system toxicity with tendency to urine infections, diarrhea and muscle weakness.

Bacillus 10 has also been useful and curative in salmonella poisoning where recovery had been very slow and in one case of debility after resection of the bowel.

In these cases, Bacillus 10 seems to be able to stir the VF into producing some symptoms that can be recognised and used to find an accurate analogue for the real case, if it does not cure on its own, as it frequently does. It enables the VF to tell you what it needs.

I have also used Bacillus 10 in patients with pain in the coccyx from falling or after anal rape, or with fatty cysts in any part of the body when there is a history of internal trauma. I have also used it successfully when Staphysagria did not work with vulval itching and fishy discharges after rape.

In girls (mainly) where anorexia results from self-loathing and self-punishment it has proved useful but, although well indicated, I have never had success in cases of deliberate self-harm such as cutting.

I have also used the remedy in some cases of gall bladder problems, ringworm and dermatitis but only where there has been some prior physical trauma to the soft parts of the internal organs.

Therapeutics

Asthma	Dermatitis	Poisoning	Pruritis

Generalities

Slow or sluggish bodily processes
Aversion to breakfast, cannot face eating in the morning
Allergies to various food substances or inhaled toxins.

Head

Headache restricted to forehead or begins in forehead.
Headache radiates to left eye. Head pains from odours.

Eyes

Sharp pain in eye or dull ache associated with head pain.

Nose

Nonspecific catarrh

Mouth and Voice

Spongy and bleeding gums and offensive, fishy breath

Back

Pain in either iliac fossa

Profuse perspiration in axillae

Sore pain in coccyx, rarely sharp.

Cysts.

Chest and Heart

Chest muscle inflammation and associated soreness.

Abdomen

Sharp pain in area of gall bladder

Rawness in body creases from perspiration

Stomach and digestion

Nausea and vomiting

Craves sweets and chocolates and fried fish

Aversion to eggs, bread, tomato and breakfast generally.

Loss of appetite

Rectum and Stool

Anal pruritis. Sluggish bowel movements. Stool passes only slowly.

Kidneys and Urinary

Frequency of urging and urination

Female

Vulval pruritis. Fishy odour. Greenish corrosive leucorrhoea.

Raw and cracked skin. Boils. Raised libido

Male

Offensive discharges from penis. Increased desire.

Sweat and raw in scrotal creases.

Respiration and lungs

Asthmatic breathing with cough < morning

Expectoration of mucous

Extremities

Sore muscles of thigh and calf, not affected by movement.

Arthritic stiffness in either knee

Skin

Tendency to warts and felons. Ringworm.

Dermatitis, cracking and rawness in flexures

General Modalities

< eggs and animal fats

Related remedies

Nux vomica   Phosphorus

Colibacillinum/ E.Coli

The keynotes for this remedy are emotional doubt and physical sepsis
There is a loss of determination, irresolution, indecisiveness and a lack of resolve or gumption.
As a character Colibacillinum may be hypercritical, extremely fastidious and afraid of dirt and disease. When sick these characteristics may exaggerate but they are usually present at least in a mild form. They are changeable to varying degrees, worse when sick.
They doubt themselves and their abilities to deal with even the most minor setbacks and they have a general and pronounced inability to cope with and form of stress. They may have obsessions about minor elements of their lives.

They micro manage their life to reduce anxiety and pressure but this leads to phobias of crowds, claustrophobia and open spaces from their desire to reduce their stress, and they suffer from general disassociation with reality. In health, they may be extremely adaptable and manage changes well, whereas in sickness they find any change troublesome, and coping with life in general becomes a struggle.
Anxiety makes them restless and they are unable to keep still or sometimes even to remain in one physical location, but anticipating travel to come makes them anxious.
Alternatively, they may simply withdraw into themselves whilst awake or seek the sanctuary of sleep.
Unless constantly with a supporter they feel abandoned and left to cope alone, which they feel unable to do, which leads to weeping. They are melancholy, gloomy and depressed.
They do not think or plan well an often describe themselves as empty headed.
There is a general loss of memory and confusion about things they used to find certainty in. They forget names, words and faces and recent events and are prone to malapropisms.

Generalities

Reckeweg uses preparation Colibacillinum for all forms of antibiotic overuse.

Symptoms of all sorts may alternate or change at frequent intervals.
Their general symptoms include hypotension and a tendency towards fainting. There is limited energy, although they feel the need to keep moving and the patients are thus worn out and weak. They are fatigued but often without apparent reason. They are very chilly especially after eating, which seems to drain them of energy adding to their frequent prostration.
There are also China-like complaints from loss of fluids or even failure to refresh the body's stores of liquid.
Chilly, especially after eating. Feverish, causing weakness.
In fevers and infections, they are prone to suffer delusions.

Head
The head feels empty and there are head pains from anxiety, contradiction, argument or in anticipation of an argument. Frontal headaches.
Eyes/ Vision
Objects seem nearer than they really are.
Mouth and Tongue
The tongue may have a yellowish / white coating or a red stripe down the centre. Unpleasant taste.
Face
The face is pale, even pallid and there is swelling of the upper eyelids and a pain behind eyes that the patient will describe as a headache. Acne roseacea.
Neck and back
Can't hold themselves erect. They lack the strength.

Abdomen

There is slow digestive transit with heaviness in the abdomen. Patients are bloated soon after eating and that distention is slow to pass. Excessive amounts of flatulence. There are abdominal spasms and heavy drawing sensations or rumbles in the abdomen. There are colic and severe but unfocussed pains originating in the gall bladder or liver.

Stomach and digestion

They may have a capricious appetite and many food items seem to cause flatus which is copious and frequently offensive but does not seem to relieve the digestion. Colibacillinum patients are aggravated by dairy, eggs and fish, most especially producing wind but also diarrhoea and headaches. Prone to food poisoning, cannot cope with even mild digestive aggravations.

Rectum and stool

There is diarrhoea of all causations or none. There may also be an alternating diarrhoea and constipation, most frequently as in one-day diarrhoea and the next day constipated.

Severe diarrhoea with dehydration. Traveller's diarrhoea.

Even when regular and without difficulty the stools are usually offensive, sometimes bloody, and there are infestations of worms that do not easily respond to conventional treatments. Flatus is loud and offensive,

Kidneys and urinary

Colibacillinum has frequency and urgency of urination passing only small amounts each time but without the ability to prevent urine escaping. The remedy has been of significant benefit in cases of irritable bladder. There is an odd urging to urinate shortly after urination. There is often a burning in urethra especially after urination and at end of flow leading to its use in cystitis, especially recurrent. There may be blood in the urine and an offensive or musty odour to it. The urine is often turgid and very yellow and there may be blood detectable in it, especially just before the cystitis symptoms appear.

Female

Julian considers Colibacillinum excellent in all pelvic inflammatory disease and inflammation especially where there is no acute attack, developing slowly and remaining at a low level of infection and/or fever.

There is bright yellow leucorrhoea which may have burning as a concomitant and there is poor libido because of vaginal and vulval discomfort and pain during penetrative sex. There are also vaginal burning sensations unconnected with intercourse. Menses are normal in quantity and quality in most cases but there may be amenorrhea. There may be inflammation throughout the reproductive system such as vaginitis and salpingitis.

Male

The male may experience a painful ejaculation but usually has a low libido. There is also a tendency to a burning pain in the urethra after sexual intercourse. The patient is prone to cystitis, prostatitis and epididymitis.

Sleep

Deep and heavy sleep leaving him barely able to function for hours after. He may also find it very difficult to get to sleep. Heavy sweating in sleep.

Extremities

Pain in small joints. Blue discolouration of joints. Coldness. Nodules in joints.

General modalities

>Heat

<Cold < humidity < seaside < after rest < exertion < dairy < eggs

Related remedies

Arsenicum alb	**China**	
Folliculinum	**Medorrhinum**	
Psorinum	**Pyrogen**	**Sepia**

Dysentery-co

The keynote for Dys-co is apprehension but that does the remedy a disservice because it is more than apprehension - its nearer to terror. Apprehension is the word that is in some of the text books, but it is almost more than a fear even, it is a certainty that something is going to go wrong. If you remember from Argentum Nit the extreme fear where they know that if they go around that next corner, someone is going to bop them on the head. This is the same certainty and it shows the symbiotic relationship between Argentum Nit and Dysentery Co.

The basic character of those who need the remedy is one that demonstrates avoidance as a basic characteristic. They tend not to put their heads above the parapet to be shot at, but avoid the responsibility and therefore the blame when things go wrong.

Although you get the general lacking in confidence, it's not so much "oh dear I don't think I could do that" but rather every time a challenge comes up, they try and avoid it because they are certain they are going to fail. The fear is an active thing for them. For most of us, a lack of confidence is wishing we didn't have to do some things and being certain we are not going to do it very well but with Dys-Co they actively work to avoid the challenge. You can certainly say they are the quintessential cowards. Dys-Co patients feel as if everything they do is wrong and is going to go even more wrong. They are hypersensitive to all criticism such that if they put the knives and forks down not quite far enough apart for the plate, and you say, could you put them slightly further apart next time, their reaction may be "I knew you didn't want me to do this, you think I am incompetent, you think I can't actually control my life".

This extreme reaction can come from really such small things. When you are dealing with someone who needs Dys-Co you should walk on egg shells the whole time because everything that you say they take as an indication of how awful they are. If you ask them to do something, then they couldn't possibly because it would go wrong - they just know it would go wrong and then you would hate them!

They are highly strung and uneasy with all new things even if they don't involve challenges. I gave Dys-Co to one patient who was a minister of religion and when he was going on holiday, he needed to scout out the place first and look at the church incognito so that when he went into the church he would know where everything was in case someone asked him to take part in the service. He always had to plan because he couldn't face being somewhere and doing something without considering and planning beforehand to try and cover all eventualities.

Dys-co is easily flustered - doing two things at once is totally impossible. You should ask them to do one thing and when they have finished, you ask them to do another thing. If you ask them to do the second one before they have finished the first one, they can't cope with the difficulty of deciding how best to perform the two tasks. They are always expecting something to go wrong, in old fashioned terms they borrow trouble. The sort of person that comes in and says I am very worried - you say why - and they say I don't know. They get flustered if someone interrupts them and then they can't possibly get back to what they were saying before - you interrupt the stream and they don't have any reference point to get back to where they were so they lose it.

Dys-co is related to Argentum Nit - experienced practitioners often use it as an acute of Argentum Nit. My experience is that it can be either way around.

Patients mainly tend to have an aversion to strangers, either with anxiety in case they are murderers or rapists, or if they should say something wrong!
Dys-co is very important in my remedy tool kit for anything to do with an inability to cope with any challenges or changes but certainly you will find an awful lot of relationships between Arg Nit and Dys Co.
The other major symptom of note of course is embarrassment. They are modest and they blush easily, use other words to denote body functions. They blush if they see someone breast feeding, must leave the room if they see a couple making love on television. There are so many challenges - they can't relax- so many things are asked of them during the day. Make supper - yes but what?
The emotional patient weeps from challenges, anxieties or excitement always the thought that something may go wrong.
When they do produce something, it is usually good because they are quite **creative** - they are talented, but they can't allow themselves to be interrupted.
I have a Dys-co patient and when she moved to a new house, the first thing that had to be done on the property, was that a shed had to be built at the bottom of the garden, not for the garden tools but as a workshop for her.
The only way that she could get anything done was to get away from the telephone, away from the front door bell so that she could work in peace and only come out when she wanted to.
There was to be no communication from the house to the garden shed because any contact disturbed what she was doing and if she was disturbed she could never get the train of activity back on the rails. If the place burnt down, I suspect her family might disturb her but otherwise probably not.

There is a tubercular desire to move or travel - I might express it as a method of escape from the creditors and the challenges. They can't cope with things that are demanded of them, so they move on - if they stay in a place, people get used to them and ask them things. If you keep moving, you stay hidden. That's the lesser of the two evils. The physical restlessness goes with that too. There is a bustle and hurry about them when they are doing anything, a restless desire to finish before something goes wrong.

They are easily knocked down into weariness and depression. They have an unforgiving energy bank manager. I find this concept of an energy bank quite a useful one to help my patients.

When they find themselves getting better but still tired, they say, "my symptoms are improving but I am still so weary". I say, well what you have done is overdrawn your energy bank and now you must pay back what you have overdrawn with interest and that is still why you are not actually feeling the benefits yet even though the symptoms have improved. They usually understand that - many have had cheques bounced by their bank and they are simply getting energy cheques bounced and they seem to respond to that quite well.
Dys Co has that unforgiving energy bank manager so the interest rates are quite high. If they give off some energy, they then must sleep a lot to get it back and you will usually find that Dys Co patients sleep a lot. One of the worst things that can happen to them is insomnia. It says in the text books, insomnia from shock. I think it could be classified as insomnia from any challenge or disturbance so not even as severe as a shock. When they do drop off to sleep, for them it is like falling from a great height so they hit the bottom and wake up again

They suffer from the classic symptom of brain fag and have a loss of train of thought if mentally stretched. There is also a fog of the brain and their thoughts may be severely confused. They are claustrophobic for places and people and especially cannot bear being too close to many people and of course a hatred of crowds.

Their feeling of failure may lead them to thoughts of suicide but their lack of courage makes it very unlikely that they would follow through. I have had several patients with suicidal thoughts but none have progressed to anything active.

Dys Co is a very good remedy for postnatal depression. They are in a state of change, they are not getting the sleep they were before, their energy is depleted - so it's not surprising they are depressed.

The condition may affect anybody, but it applies doubly to Dys Co because they have so few resources to spare. They are also worried that they are going to do some harm to their baby by not being able to 'do' it right. You have never seen so many baby books as a Dys Co patient will have. Then of course what happens is you read all these baby books and they don't all say the same thing so they panic because do they follow Dr Spock or Dr Miriam Stoppard? I mean personally I am inclined to the bigger tome - by the time you have looked up "blue, baby turning of" in the index - the baby has turned pink again, so you leave well alone. It doesn't always happen like that of course because if you are a Dys Co, you cannot help it. You know that something is going to get worse - it's an awful state to be in - it's a real panic at small problems.

They are afraid when events are beyond their control, public transport is especially bad for them, and in large groups of people. There are many fears including the future and of the dark and the unknown.

Overall you are looking at an excessively sensitive and over reactive individual, so anxiety and fear never really leave them alone. They are always concerned about something and what you the homoeopath can deal with, is the level at which they are operating so if 'normal' is at one floor, a lot of the time they are 20 floors higher and are just 'normal' a little of the time. If you give them Dys Co you shift all that down about five floors or even more, so they are just panicking occasionally which is an awful lot of improvement.

So, anything is an ordeal. Leaving home to go to work - leaving home to take the baby for a walk - what if I have forgotten something.

There is a wonderful piece that could be about Dys Co in a Peanuts cartoon strip some years ago - Charlie Brown says to Linus "I thought you were going on holiday"? "Well we were" says Linus "but Mum got worried". She says "What happens if we were driving along the freeway at 70 miles an hour and something went wrong with the glove compartment". This rather sums up how easy it is for the Dys-co to get panicked. Many things which the rest of us would smile at is a worry for them. You will often find them making lists - you often have a little list stuck by the door. Have you done this, this and this? Have you put the keys here? Have you locked all the back doors?

When they stop doing things, then they start thinking about doing things - so the worse time for them is when they are ready to go to sleep because they can't be distracted by having to do something, so they now have plenty of time to think about things. They panic about what they have done, and they panic about what they have got to do tomorrow so the sign on the door says, if all else fails, panic.

I think this is sycotic - it has syphilitic tendencies because all of this is self-harming to them but it's mainly sycotic - over reaction constantly.

Dys-co gets palpitations from stress and anxiety. There is air hunger - they crave air, crave warmth. They are very chilly individuals because everything is constantly moving - their brain is constantly active. Their thinking uses up more calories than going to the gym. I have great difficulty convincing people of this.

With all this stressful activity, they are fidgety and twitchy and they are aggravated by all the things that cause them to be fidgety and twitchy. They are aggravated by excitement and any form of stimulation. Their sex life tends to be non-existent because they might do it wrong. If they didn't do it wrong, they would probably catch something. The worst case - they would probably do something wrong and catch something. So Dys-co is not a happy bunny.

Generalities

The pain that they feel is sometimes out of proportion to the perception of the practitioner as to the seriousness of the condition, so they seem to suffer more than you would expect them to do. They are very sensitive to pain.

Dys-co are anemic, pallid and puffy.

They feel lousy all the time - the worst time is usually 3am to 6am. From my point of view, they are anxious all the time but certainly 3am to 6am - it's the middle of the night - they are the only one awake and it's an obvious time to be anxious.

Dys-co desires warmth but is easily overheated when she has to seek open air to relieve it, but soon gets chilly and needs warmth yet again.

Easily exhausted by stress or anxiety and the excitement produces symptoms in the physical body.

Dys-co makes involuntary movements, particularly when anxious and everyone will usually have at least one involuntary reaction to sudden excitement or stress ranging from blushing or facial tics to twitches of the limbs or involuntary flatus. Finds it difficult to stay still. Fidgets constantly, which is associated with a feeling of constriction.

One of their classic symptoms is the tendency to feel as if there were lumps, plugs or blockages in individual organs.

Head

The scalp is painful with or without head pain and there is a tendency to dandruff.

There are cyclical headaches - cyclical migraines - headaches relieved by vomiting but worse after sleep. Also, headaches aggravated by strain, excitement, anxiety, heat or stuffiness, which are sometimes described as a fuzzy head. The cycle of these headaches may be related to hormonal changes but this is not always the case. Sometimes the patient can identify a causation or a rhythm but often we can only utilize the remedy when the description is 'regular' with no qualifiers. Their eyeballs frequently get tender with the headache.

Eyes

Eyeballs feel sore with headache. Styes. Blepharitis. Conjunctivitis with photophobia. Infections can have a long prodromal period. Floaters with disturbed or discoloured vision.

Ears

Hearing reduces when tinnitus sounds appear or increase. Hot discharges when infected. They may feel as if their heartbeat is in their ears.

Nose

Hay fever. Frequent coryza. Pain at the root of the nose. Rhinorrhoea.

Mouth and Voice
Tongue raw, burning and dry or coated. Taste burnt or foul. Prone to stammering.
Face
Pallid and puffy. Facial tics and twitches when under stress. Quivering small muscles, especially in eyelids. There is acne roseacea which may be aggravated by overindulgence in sugary sweets. Lips cracked and dry and bluish.
Orbital or trigeminal neuralgias.
Throat
Dry, sore throats and recurrent tonsillitis. Swollen or merely atrophied thyroid.
Thyrotoxicosis. Hay fever with dry swelling internally.
Chest and Heart
The heart can be felt pounding in the ears. Palpitations on waking and before events.
Chest pains on exertion and tight muscles sore.
They suffer from tachycardia, with constrictive pains around the chest
Back
General rheumatic pain and stiffness. Spondylitis.
Respiration and lungs
Dys-co has asthma from anxiety which you would expect, together with palpitations from anxiety, tachycardia, constrictive pains around the chest and if you get that what have you got - well its bound to be a heart attack they think. They believe they are bound to be going to die because if you get the slightest thing - it's always going to be worse with these patients.
Breathlessness on waking with anxiety.
There is bronchial cataarh, dullness and thickening of the lungs and bloody sputum and a nervous cough associated with anxiety.
Pleurodynia.

Stomach and digestion

All anxieties manifest as stomach discomfort and almost any stomach or abdominal pain can need Dys-co.

There is an almost permanent indigestion together with a digestive pain relieved by eating. This can mimic duodenal ulcer pains or Gastro-oesophageal Reflux Disease.

An empty feeling in the stomach relieved briefly by eating or lying down. There may also be pain aggravated by eating which may lead to loss of appetite.

There is an emptiness or nausea between meals and eating often ameliorates briefly.

There is heartburn that materializes hours after eating and acrid or bilious water brash.

Dys-co has a desire for cold drinks which nevertheless often aggravate together with sweet things and animal fats which also often aggravate (although often because of overconsumption as they don't know when to stop!)

Their digestion is so poor that despite eating good food they may become emaciated.

Abdomen

The pains in the abdomen all are sometimes improved by urination. Colitis. Colic.

Like Arg Nit this is a very windy remedy - they get flatus from anxiety - it's nothing to do with food - and it can happen at any time, day or night, from anxiety, and can be painful as well as distending the abdomen. There may be an inability to release trapped wind. Gall bladder area is tender to touch or from tight clothing.

Male

Masturbation frequent in very young boys.

Female

Thinks she will die from menstrual pain.

Irregular menses. Throbbing pain on perineum.

Tendency to frequent masturbation.

Fibroids.

Rectum and Stool

Stools tend to be frequently loose without being diarrhoea and they also suffer from irritable bowel syndrome - aggravated by any challenges or anxieties of course. Diarrhoea during headache. There is colitis from stress – she is sure she has bowel cancer.

You need to keep re-assuring them. In this they are like Phosphorus - they will believe you until you have gone out of the room, so you must keep re-assuring them.

Dys-co may have a throbbing or pulsing sensation in the rectum but when they try to pass a stool there feels as if there is a blockage preventing expulsion.

They may also have many loose stools during a day and stools tend to be forcible just like the explosive Sulphur stool. They may also be dry, knotted and difficult to expel from weakness of the muscle.

The trouble with the forcible stools is that the patients often have anal fissures so that stooling is uncomfortable too. You can also get difficult expulsion of the stool and that is more commonly associated with the anal fissures.

The weakness is probably because of fear of the pain from trying to expel the stool, so they lose the ability to push.

You have got the alternation here, the forcible stools and the frequent stools or you have got the difficulty in letting the stool go, which is usually associated with problems with the sphincter and cracks in the sphincter.

The concomitant is mostly fear, fear with everything.

Any complaint is worse than it seems to be to the practitioner.

Piles that protrude and are aggravated by motion.

Kidneys and Urinary

Dys-co has difficulty in holding on to their urine. They are worse for moving about and urinate at least twice as often away from home. Movement in a vehicle causes urging to urinate. Every time they see a loo they must visit it when they are away from home in case there isn't one where they are going to be in ten minutes' time when they do want to go. That is not to do with the need to urinate - it's the anxiety that they might need to urinate. If you keep on doing that, you create the condition you are trying to avoid so you create problems by the frequency of your urination.

Enuresis when anxious, especially in boys.

Sleep and dreams

Too many thoughts to sleep, mostly anxious and stressful. Starting in sleep causing waking in panic.

Falling sensation on dropping off to sleep, which wakes them.

Wakes with anxiety and abdominal pains 2 to 3 am.

Extremities

Pain in joints.

Skin

They have oily skins and warts. There are hanging warts with stalks but not like fig-wart disease, just the stalks alone.

Hard skin and callouses form easily

General Modalities

<: 3am to 6 am

>: urination

Related remedies

Anacardium
Arsenicum Alb
Argentum Nit
Carcinosin
Lycopodium
Nux Vomica
Veratrum Alb

Faecalis

This is one of the lesser used bowel nosodes, even in my own clinic. Nevertheless, it does have some clear symptoms and can be useful in specific circumstances.

The keynote symptoms here are a lack of flexibility, mental, emotional and physical, as well as overall sluggishness.

Faecalis patients are not those we usually look forward to seeing in our clinics. They are difficult to shift from their life stance and behaviours, slow to take up opportunities for improvement in life or in health and reluctant to accept that you are offering them worthwhile options. They are concerned about, and impatient with change and slow to shift opinions that have become fixed, regarding possible options for change as not worth the effort.
They have become insular, and are unwilling to make any allowance for others and often begin to dislike even those they are close to. I am reluctant to use the phrase 'loved ones' here as they really do not have much love left over for anyone other than themselves. They are self-obsessed and the only way to persuade them of something is to emphasise the benefit to themselves. Even then, because of their aversion to change, they may not hold to decisions they seem to have made!

They are slow to express specific emotions, being suppressed in that area. They show general irritability and unfocussed anger with no fine shades of behaviour. They do seem to weep easily, most usually when talking about their own problems, but are still unable to give individualizing symptoms which are easily prescribable.

They are weary both mentally and physically and limited in movement as well as intellect.

Physically these patients are worse for over consumption of fat and sugar, especially producing liverish or bilious symptoms as a result. Their digestive symptoms seem to indicate an excess of acid and are often exemplified by acid reflux and nausea.

They tend to be chilly and to have noticeable cold spots around the body, most especially the digestive organs and the extremities. They need sleep which does not seem to refresh them. Overheating is always bad and they may be flushed if ill. Skin problems are aggravated by heat.

Digestive transit is very slow and elimination of stool is difficult, though the stool itself is not usually hard. Haemorrhoids are frequently present though they do not usually bleed of their own accord.
Digestive pains are felt as severe as are menstrual pains. The menopause seems to increase frequency and severity of pain.
It has often been helpful in treatment of type 2 Diabetes.

Complaints that indicate a need for Faecalis tend to come on slowly, as if even their Vital Force rejects change, develop slowly and take time to reach their ultimation. The underfunction of the Vital Force seems here to work to the patient's benefit, slowing the damage. It is often necessary to repeat Faecalis several times to maintain any improvement.

Related remedies

Bacillus #7   Sepia

Gaertner

The keynote with Gaertner is mal absorption.

That instantly makes us think about Coeliac disease, Crohn's disease, IBS, failure to thrive in children together with allergies and sensitivities to food because what is an allergy except a failure to absorb something- a failure of the body to deal with something. There are a lot of allergic responses with this remedy. It is most frequently given to children of course, whose development is slow or poor but I use it in adults quite regularly as well. Mostly the adults tend to get it after being affected by too much antibiotic treatment or because of allergies or failure to recover from a debilitating disease. So, in that sense it's not so much a failure to absorb but a failure to bounce back. You can see why the appearance is generally thought of as emaciated.

Malabsorption, allergies and antibiotic poisoning all reduce the immune system's ability to defend itself and thus many symptoms that belong to no obvious syndrome can be produced.

Let's move on to mental and emotional symptoms. These apply to adults and children but are more obvious in children. Children don't conceal things quite as well as adults do. We start off by looking at hypersensitivity. As well as finding it difficult to absorb things through the gut, they find it difficult to absorb and dispel emotional trauma.

In other words, they are like an open book. If you say something which wounds them, you can see the results in their expression. That might be very satisfying if you are of an evil taint. Gaertner patients are hypersensitive to insults and to changes in atmosphere, both emotional and physical.

Because of their difficulty of adaption (and remember you are still thinking in terms of the Calc carb type syndrome here) they are nervous, anxious and are aware of their own sensitivity.

When these traumas happen to them, they find it difficult to let go of the emotions so they are made miserable by them and their results. They become pessimistic. What's the point of doing something if somebody is always going to put me down for it? Still because of this difficulty in absorption which we for the purposes of the lecture, will interpret as a failure to adjust, then they are also afraid of the dark, the unknown and afraid of new things. This also goes for their diet of course because they are afraid to try new things in case the new food upsets them. They like routine, physically and emotionally and are uneasy and restless in case something goes wrong.

They find it difficult to settle until whatever is going to happen has happened. They don't maintain concentration. This is where the difference comes in with the carbonates. You can put Calc carb down in front of a puzzle and it will play quite happily for hours even if it has only used a few pieces. Gaertner children don't have that ability to concentrate so they are restless mentally, inquisitive but lacking in concentration. Their attention span is a problem and I have used the remedy in attention deficit disorder which is one of the major childhood diseases that we see. Some of those cases that we see may not be ADD or ADHD but whatever the diagnosis they often respond to Gaertner. You have seen the sort of thing, you tell the child to go and look at a book and they do so for about 30 seconds and then want to do something else. We used to call it boredom.

These patients are disruptive - they don't do what they are told - you can't rely on them. Attention deficit disorder is typical Gaertner and you can see that, very often, these are children who are supposed to have allergies anyway and the treatment involved, if the parents are in any way, shape or form alternative, is to start withdrawing colourants and those sorts of things. I have found sometimes that you can short circuit that by giving Gaertner and they improve significantly without changing the diet. Sometimes it means you only should get rid of one thing as opposed to half their food intake which is what you may have to do if you rely on allergy tests.

Although they don't always stay with what they have been told to do they are eager to please and want your approval- the problem is always that they simply cannot remain still physically or mentally for very long.

They like security, they like to know there is something to hold on to, someone to hold on to and they do not like sleeping alone, sometimes they simply won't sleep alone.

One other thing which is odd, just going back to the fear of being alone, they have a fear of dark like Calc Carb but they may also love the dark. I had one little Gaertner boy who used to go around turning all the lights off. There was a light outside in the street and he liked the flickering from that and he didn't mind the flickering of the television - he didn't like having any extra light. He went away with Gaertner but I was sure there was something else underlying it but he never came back so I presumed he was better.

We should add different things with adults but yes, I had one adult who used to sleep with the light on and he was in his forties and he would always sleep with a light on when he was alone. He was fine when there was someone else in the house, didn't even have to be in the same room, but otherwise he always needed the light on.

Gaertner patients only have a limited number of foods they really like. As with Calc Carb, they might very well exist on three things for ages until the fancy strikes them to add number four. They are very faddy eaters.

During sleep, they do have the night terrors as well that you get in Calc. carb. or Phosphorus but they also sleep walk. I had one case where the child would come downstairs, have a conversation and go back up to bed, whilst still asleep - the child was about 9. During the night, especially with the terrors they sweat a lot. There is a severe fear of dark and gloomy places. Fear of being alone.
Therapeutically, we use Gaertner for antibiotic poisoning. I lose track of the number of times that I give Gaertner in cases where children have been given huge doses of antibiotics. Sometimes you get a child who has had a dozen course of antibiotics in a year - it almost doesn't matter what the original symptom was at that point - you have got to give them something to get over the effect of the antibiotics. This is especially true for non-penicillin based antibiotics.

This can even work many years later. You might have to give it at a higher potency but I had one case of never been well since some illness which I can't remember now but the child had two years of antibiotics until they gave up and said well he has got this low-grade infection. We could give him the antibiotic all the rest of his life but it is not getting any worse - its staying at this level and I suggest we leave it.

He had this for two or three more years and then they brought him to me and I gave him Gaertner not for the original condition but for the antibiotics and of course the original condition came back and went away without further treatment. Sometimes it does that because what the antibiotics did is prevent the resolution of the problem.

You can use Gaertner for antibiotic poisoning now, or in the past, or even if they seemed to cure the condition that was there originally. Sometimes it cures the condition that was there originally, sometimes it cures the antibiotic poisoning, sometimes it cures the whole shooting match. It is an extraordinarily powerful remedy. Whenever I see recurrent courses of antibiotics, the file opens at Gaertner. I have to try and stop myself giving Gaertner automatically as I have done it so often. Therapeutically for allergies - where there is strong and compelling evidence that the patient is worse from some foods particularly to starchy grains.

So obviously, it is going to be a remedy for bowel problems like Crohn's Disease and colitis and IBS and a very good remedy after surgical interventions to any of those areas. It is great for surgical interventions to the gut or even to the stomach.

Gaertner is a major remedy for biting nails. (Often anxiety of course) and for ear discharges, ear infections, throat and chest infections and of course those are some of the things that get treated by antibiotics. The only sorts of infections which have never needed Gaertner in my practice are those of the urinary tract (often Sycotic-co or Colibac) and skin infections (often Morgan Pure).

The patient may have styes or, especially, mouth ulcers that don't heal or keep recurring, not so much the ones that come and go but the ones that come and hang around being a nuisance for ages. There is also herpes of the lips, cold sores, fissured tongue, blackened teeth, nasal polyps and of course catarrh. What happens to the catarrh? It becomes infected and you get post nasal drip and it goes down and it becomes infected - so what happens when you get infected? You get antibiotics! The sequence is very predictable.

Many of the conditions for which you might be given antibiotics as a child fit the symptom picture of Gaertner anyway. It is the infection link breaker. What I am keen to point out to you is that it's not just because we know it has this effect on antibiotics but because it matches the conditions the antibiotics were prescribed for in the first place. That satisfies me because I don't like giving things by rote.

Patients are slow to recover and this is a general indication for Gaertner - which is another reason why they may have been given antibiotics.

Generalities

Numbness

Periodicity or relapsing complaints

Emaciated or flabby. Restlessness and sensitivity, physical and mental. Slow development.

They might get suppuration from the skin at the same time as they have a bowel problem or they might get infected nasal discharges at the same time as they have ear ache so there is often suppuration or cysts. What that is implying is that there is a problem throughout the whole body rather than a problem in one specific area. Gaertner is a remedy which does affect the whole of the system - I can't recommend it highly enough to you - it is an important remedy for all those things.

Head

Headache associated with digestive upsets or too many sweets. Cluster headaches.

Eyes

Tendency to styes. Spots and flickers in vision.

Ears

Tendency to infections especially in teething children

Nose

Thick and sticky cataarh, difficult to expel. Nasal polyps.

Mouth and Voice

Tongue cracked. Dark discolouration on teeth. Soft teeth. Too much saliva.

Face

Herpes. Dry scaly eruptions. Tinea Barba.

Throat

Sticky mucous causes need to scrape. Acid water brash in throat.

Back

Hip, lumbar and back pains with stiffness

Chest and Heart

Circinate eruptions on chest. Atrophy of mammae. Cysts or nodules in mammae.

Abdomen

Gall stone colic. Acid pains. Distention.

Stomach and digestion

They have gastro-intestinal symptoms and may vomit everything back that they eat. They feel their emotions in the stomach just like Kali Carb often do. They also have pains in the stomach associated with other complaints. Unable to digest fats. Malnourished even where the diet is reasonable. Weak/poor digestion. Acid eructation. Tendency to food allergies.

Frequent gastro-enteritis. Vomiting of any food, especially after too many sweets.

Desires oats, dairy products, sweet things

Averse bread, meat, fish and shellfish

Rectum and Stool

Constipation with difficult expulsion of stool. Offensive diarrhoea. Bloody discharges. Anal pruritis. Tendency to worms. There is constipation or diarrhoea with blood and/or mucus in the stool and the constipation or diarrhoea tends to happen in well-defined bouts. The patient may have one symptom and follow it with the other - or they have one and then they are normal and then they have it again so it's a rhythmic bowel complaint. Tendency to all types of worm infestations. Foul odour to stools and flatus.

Kidneys and Urinary

Blood and mucous in the urine. Burning pain in the urethra. Night time enuresis. Frequent urging or involuntary urination, worse at night.

Female

Females may have vulvar pruritis - itching of the vulva and offensive, infected leucorrhoea that needs treatment by antibiotics – which means more Gaertner needed. Vaginal itching.

Male

Hydrocele. Scrotal swellings. Boils and cysts on scrotum.

Respiration and lungs

Snoring. Bronchitis with slow recovery. Coughs at night only. Noisy breathing.

Sleep and dreams

Snoring. Cannot, or will not, sleep without light or company.

Walks in sleep. Nightmares.

Extremities

I have already mentioned nail biting, both as a habit and from anxiety. There are chilblains and muscle pains not associated with exercise. As a concomitant, something that you look for in the history particularly is infection associated with complaints, sometimes in a remote area to the original problem.

Skin
Perspiration in bed. Urticaria.
Tendency to boils or cysts.
They have circular eruptions - have you come across these wonderful circles of eruptions on chest and thighs that look like ringworm. Calc. Carb. has them a lot - in Gaertner they are mainly on the chest and you know when they are getting better, because they gradually get bigger and bigger and gaps appear in the ring until they just fade away.
General Modalities
< eating animal fats < sweets < cold and stormy weather

Related remedies

Calc. Carb	Calc. Fluor	Calc. Phos	Kali. Phos
Merc	Phos	Phyt	Puls
Sil	Tub	Zinc	

Morgan-Bach

Morgan-Bach is the compound from which Morgan-Gaertner and Morgan-Pure were isolated. It is included in this Materia Medica as some practitioners, though not myself, prefer to use the entire compound remedy rather than the individual ones.

Just as with Morgan-Pure, the main keynote here is congestion.

This is reflected in the way emotions can eat away at the patient. They are introspective, anxious and worried. They tend to keep themselves to themselves to concentrate on their own problems. Unfortunately, being alone means that there is no one to interrupt their gloomy reveries. They worry especially about their health and cannot escape their problems which makes them depressed even to the extent of having suicidal thoughts.

Hypertension.

Menopause

There are congestive headaches with flushing of the face, which are worse for becoming heated or for an excessively warm atmosphere, or heavy thundery weather. Headaches are also worse for stress, excitement or rocking motion as of a train or boat. Headaches may be relieved by vomiting bilious mucous. There is vertigo associated with hypertension.

The digestive tract is congested with overproduction of mucous. This may cause choking on rising, heartburn, acid reflux, and coated tongue. The whole system is sluggish with constipation, haemorrhoids and piles quite common. During the menopause, there are frequent bilious attacks or acidic eructations.

There are gallstones, with severe colic and cholecystitis and griping pains in the hepatic region.

As with Morgan-Pure there is nasal and bronchial congestion and pneumonia.

During the menopause, the whole system is flushed and congested with ovarian pains.

There is a serious tendency to haemorrhoids and varicose veins, chilblains and subjective blueness of extremities, with or without heart complaints.

Arthritis affects many joints with swelling and congestion but the knees are most frequently affected.

Most of the skin symptoms of Morgan-Pure are also seen in the compound Morgan-Bach. There are many symptoms in all areas and of all types including herpes, boils, fissures, eczema, impetigo, acne, dermatitis, prickly heat and erysipelas. Eruptions of all types but most frequently raw and discharging. Severe itching. The skin is dry and cracks particularly on the face, around the mouth and on the cheeks.

Morgan-Gaertner

Biliousness runs throughout the remedy Morgan Gaertner.

What sort of mind symptoms are you going to be expecting from someone like that?

They tend to be very critical, pernickety and censorious and to always be picking holes in things and people, finding the small holes in logic, action and belief that others would allow to pass. Morgan Gaertner is acid in its' responses to people and behaviour, not allowing leeway to anyone in their expressed thoughts or actions. They tend to be blunt and unnecessarily cruel, making no allowances for others and things must be done in their time frame. They are very impatient and continually restless.

Their anger is quick and strong but not as violent as others, being more like extreme irritability than violence and their anxiety is of the same ilk being grumbling rather than overpowering. The anxiety is worse when they have no-one to take the pressure from them or when there are challenges ahead of them including interacting with others, especially those who might have more technical expertise than themselves. They mostly prefer to be with people if they are the dominant ego in that company. They do like people to be subservient to them and are jealous of others success and envious of their possessions. When there is nothing else to worry about they are likely to be anxious about their health, especially as they are very limited in their trust of health professionals.

They are prone to anticipatory anxiety as well as being anxious in crowds or when physically or emotionally hemmed in. as when they are being pressured either intellectually or emotionally.

They are uncomfortable being with someone as intellectual or knowledgeable as they are and feel the pressure of reduced physical space as in claustrophobia and reduced wriggle room in arguments.
Surprisingly they like to hold and be held by another person.
The Morgan Gaertner patient cannot bear his own suffering and feels that he does not deserve it. In extremis, he will shout and cry out, having no vestige of self-control, no 'stiff upper lip'. He even cries out in his sleep from nightmares. He also is prone to overreacting at others traumas and may seem to be emotionally caring where, in truth, it is simply a reaction to an emotional stimulus. They moan and complain about life in general as well as their own suffering.
Generally, Morgan Gaertner is worse for excitement and in company.
You will certainly gather from all the above that Morgan Gaertner patients are self-absorbed and indeed, self-pitying because they are the centre of their own universe and detached from everyone else's.
Morgan Gaertner is so very similar in a lot of symptoms to Lycopodium. They both have ear infections, sweaty feet and insomnia but the differences are notable and it's just the differences I am going to give you. Whereas the Morgan Pure is aggravated in the typical syphillitic way, night and first thing in the morning, then the aggravation time for Morgan Gaertner is **4 - 8** just like Lycopodium. You can feel the shade of Lycopodium through all the various symptoms.

Generalities

There is a physical feeling of constriction to go with the emotional. They have offensive, brown and corrosive discharges. There are one sided complaints.
There is a general physical oversensitivity, a tendency to polyps and to being undernourished.

Head
Alopecia with painful scalp. Hair loss in patches.
Congestive migraines. Mastoiditis.
Cracked scalp.
Eyes
Blepharitis, styes and corneal ulcers. Opacity of vision
Ears
Otitis, mastoiditis and boils
Buzzing sounds
Nose
Sinus infections with overproduction of mucous.
Crusty ulceration. Herpes, rhinitis.
Persistent nosebleeds often caused by hard mucous.
Nasal polyps. Post nasal catarrh.
Mouth and Voice
Bitter taste in mouth. Inflamed gums, bad breath, cracks in corner of mouth.
Sticky saliva. Tongue cracked and dirty with prickling sensation. Swollen uvula
Face
Oedematous. Left sided trigeminal neuralgia.
Left sided herpetic eruptions.
Inflamed eyelids.
Florid or pale face. Acne. Cysts. Tinea barba.
Throat
Tonsillitis. Burning or acid sensations. Sensation as if choking.
Neck and Back
Stiff neck. Fibrositis. Spondylitis.
Pain under or around right scapula.
Chest and Heart
Palpitations in the night that wake him from sleep, better for eructation of air or moving around. Angina.
Constricted pain in the chest extending to left arm.
Intercostal neuralgia.
Cold or heavy feeling sensation in chest.

Constriction or oppression.
Restless feeling in chest.
Warts on the breasts, especially thin stalks on nipples.

Abdomen

Abdominal and inguinal pain and distention. Gall stone colic. Borborygmus. Heartburn.
Incarcerated flatus. Sensation of fullness without having eaten.

Stomach and digestion

In Morgan Pure you have water brash and heartburn, whereas in Morgan Gaertner you have water brash and eructations. You can have foul smelling eructations which are empty, or eructations of bile or eructations of acid fluid. It is difficult and slow for them to digest food. Morgan Gaertner is also an important remedy for the treatment of GORD (gastro oesophageal reflux disease) which leads to many failed prescriptions for proton pump inhibitors.
Worse after eating- he may vomit after food. Abdomen distended or drowsy after eating. Indigestion from eating anything.
Craves hot (temperature) food, sweets, salt things, fats, eggs and meat. May also be averse to fat, eggs and meat.

Intestines, Rectum and Stool

Hard dry stools that are difficult to expel.
Mucosal discharges from anus.
Rectal prolapse, anal fissures.
Itchy painful and bleeding piles.
Urgent diarrhoea. Weak sphincter.
Parasites or worms are a tendency.

Kidneys and Urinary

Calculi. Kidney pains. Nephritis. Pyelitis.
Bladder pains with frequency of urination. Copious burning urine.
Night time urging and incontinence. Cystitis.
Strong odour to urine and sediment on settling.

Male

Incomplete erections. Impotence.

Female

Warts on the breasts, especially nipples.

Dysmenorrhoea. Thick brown, corrosive leucorrhoea which burns the labia. Vulvar pruritis.

Ovarian pains. Pre-Menstrual Syndrome

Respiration and lungs

Dyspnoea. Asthma. Peritonitis. Pleurodynia.

Tickling cough at night or on rising and when tired., better sitting, worse climbing stairs or lying down.

Extremities

Bites nails. Painful joints.

Hot feet at night whether or not in bed.

One side warmer than the other.

Blue discolouration of extremities.

Flat warts on hands. Large jagged warts.

Sleep

Anxious dreams of conflict.

Difficult to sleep. Cries out in sleep.

Skin

Psoriasis, eczema, urticaria, herpes. Contact dermatitis.

Warts. Cysts.

General Modalities

< 4-8 AM OR PM, company, after eating, before menses, night, heat of the bed

>Gentle motion, passing wind

Related remedies

Lycopodium	Chelidonium	Natrum Mur
Nux Vomica	Pulsatilla	Silica

Morgan Pure

The peg on which we can hang many of the symptoms of Morgan Pure is **congestion**.

We can have congestion in both the mental and physical spheres of our patients.

We see underactive and psoric depressions where there are too many alternatives for the patient to decide on a course of action, so nothing is done and they withdraw from purposeful activity. We can also see under functioning sycosis here too where the urge to activity is present but the focus allowing that activity remains elusive. Introspection and navel gazing become a substitute for involvement in the world and its' activities and gloom becomes the overarching emotion. It is as if the active emotions of happiness, pleasure and the like are unable to breach the barrier created by the emotional congestion.

They are not very stable people- it is quite easy to push them into this gloom. As people, they have difficulty in communicating both words and feelings. They let you know that things are not right without explanation of the specifics and make you suffer if possible, although your suffering and anxiety does not seem to ameliorate theirs. They are deeply anxious and want you to know about it even if they don't really expect you to be able to help them. Their anxieties are especially focused on their health and wellbeing, having a fear of dread diseases and that all sorts of innocuous foods and drinks will do them harm. (It is of course difficult to separate this irrational fear from the extremely rational one of the harm caused by certain elements of our modern diet!)

I had one patient who was given Morgan Pure whose aetiology was that as an insurance broker he had a new type of policy – to insure against dread diseases. As a result of selling this new product he could not stop thinking about dread diseases. That is typical of Morgan Pure -think of it once and then you can't stop. Morgan Pure even has a fear of crowds and of being caught up in a crowd (congestion again) and will avoid busy places to protect himself, even changing his lifestyle to accommodate his fear, going to the supermarket late at night or even ordering online for home delivery.

The anxieties build in him if he lacks an outlet (as in another person to take some of the load) and can result in suicidal impulses if left to his own devices for too long. Happily though the impulses rarely are translated into action as the turgidity of their vital force will not allow the thought to manifest into action.

He may have phobias apart from his health, the most common being agoraphobia or claustrophobia as well as the previously mentioned anthropophobia. He also has a fear of the unknown and the dark as well as new places. There is a difficulty in disposing of or acting on thoughts and urges as well as a general difficulty in making efficient communication. He is a passive depressive who cannot relieve his stresses, although he is often fruitlessly active and restless.

Everything in his mental and emotional state is worse when he is alone, although you may also find an aversion to company in the same person.

Overall the mental and emotional picture of the remedy is one of a lack of incisiveness and a tendency to dwell on disagreeable thoughts.

Generalities

Therapeutically Morgan Pure is specifically indicated when complaints appear to have been caused or aggravated by treatment from Penicillin and its' derivatives as well as by old fashioned Sulphonamides. Where complaints are concomitants of high blood pressure Morgan Pure will often relieve both problems. It is especially useful in gout, vertigo and periodic headaches.

Other conditions where Morgan Pure is indicated when symptoms match are stroke, thrombosis, varicose veins, general liver and gall bladder dysfunction as well as gallstones and kidney stones. Jaundice. Phlebitis Congestion. Complaints after penicillin.

In the physical sphere, there is congestion everywhere in the symptoms. All bodily systems are prone to becoming engorged and sluggish. The general excretive power is low, nothing flows smoothly or quickly enough.

They sleep into an aggravation.

Hypertension. Varicosity. Emaciation.

Head

Alopecia with scalp sensitivity. Scaly or weeping eruptions, especially at margins of hair.

Migraine – there are two important things with the migraine symptoms of Morgan Pure. The first one is periodicity and that is usually weekly but not always the same time - not always a week-end migraine as it might be in Iris or Nux v but it is usually once a week related to some other rhythm which we have not discovered. Usually it has a concomitant of acid eructations, water brash or some other stomach disorder - so it is classified under headaches with unspecified digestive problems.

The headaches are also worse for any form of travelling and in the extreme case, it can be worse from moving from one side to the other but mostly from place to place. This means that if you have a headache in your office you may be worse for going home - you need to stay there until it has gone and then you will be OK. It's not just motion - it's going from one point to another - so its travel over a period. I don't think it's as simple as motion because if you move your head around that does not aggravate it – it is moving from place to place.
Headaches are also worse for raised barometric pressure, any excitement or change. Frontal, occipital or vertex headache.
Head pains worse when cutting hair. Heaviness of the head.

Eyes

Conjunctivitis. Iritis. Cysts and styes.
Floaters and spots in vision.

Ears

Infected ears, offensive discharges from their ears.
Eczema inside ears. Illusory noises.
Tinnitus. Catarrhal deafness. Meniere's disease.

Nose

Sinuses congested and infected. Thin white and post nasal catarrh. Dryness of mucous membranes.
Epistaxis.
Lost or reduced sense of smell.

Mouth and Voice

Dirty tongue and offensive breath. Excess of saliva. Bad taste in mouth. Bitter or acrid taste or simply altered.
Tongue slimy, coated and swollen or feels dry.
Warts on the tongue

Face

There is unusual hair growth on the face in females and children.

He looks as if he has a headache, with florid face and wrinkled brow. Puffiness and floridity. Acne rosacea. Eczema in cracks. Erysipelas. Weeping eruptions. Cracks in corners of lips. Granular eyelids. Dryness of lips.

Throat

Morgan Pure is a cardinal remedy for any inflammatory response to infection (where Penicillin derivatives are often the medical drugs of choice) especially tonsillitis both new and recurrent with easy choking and the throat feeling constricted, blocked and lumpy inside.

Cheesy exudate from tonsils. Mucous accumulates when lying down.

As if an apple core were lodged in the throat.

Thyroid swelling and generally underactive thyroid are also part of the picture.

Neck and Back

Post herpetic neuralgia

Profuse perspiration in axillae. General stiffness of back and neck. Torticollis.

Boils and carbuncles.

Chest and Heart

Angina. Myocarditis. Palpitations.

Shingles pain.

Atrophy of mammae. Itchy breasts and nipples.

Abdomen

There may be a weeping and raw umbilicus, often with a bad odour.

Epigastric pains. Pains all over abdomen, often from incarcerated flatus.

Congestion of the liver.

Gallstone colic. Jaundice.

Stomach and digestion

Desires fats, sweets, eggs and butter. Worse from eggs and fats. May also avoid eggs and fat.

Burning pains from acid. Duodenal or peptic ulcers. Gastro-oesophageal reflux disease. Heartburn, water brash, general biliousness. Vomiting, nausea.
Sinking feeling at 11am.

Intestines, Rectum and Stool

There are piles and anal fissures which you might expect with their general sluggishness.
Many Morgan Pure patients must get up from the table to pass a stool when they begin to eat. This is a real keynote indication for Morgan Pure and I have never known it to fail with this symptom in the case.
Mucous or bloody discharge from anus.
Constipation or loose, foul smelling urgent stools. Has little control over his bowel.
Itching of anus. Piles bleed, itch and are painful and protrude.
Worms.

Kidneys and Urinary

There may be cystitis -with both frequency and pain but you probably would not be giving it unless there were other indications. The urine itself is very smelly, very offensive and corrosive. The patient can have raw patches around the urethra as compared with some of the other cystitis remedies where it hurts but you can see no reason why -with this remedy you can see a reason for the pains. Sugar in the urine.
Strong smelling urine. Enuresis in adults.

Male

Eruptions on the genitals

Female

Ovarian pains, fibroids, polyps and corrosive leucorrhoea where the symptoms match the general Morgan Pure tendencies. Brown or green discharges. Pruritis. Boils. Cysts. Menorrhagia and metrorrhagia. Bartholinitis. Pain during coition.

Respiration and lungs

There is an asthmatic tendency, and the remedy is extremely effective in many patients where respiratory complaints alternate with skin complaints. You will also often find an 'unholy trinity' of respiration, digestion and eruption, all causing problems in the same patient at different times.

Asthma, Emphysema. Pleurodynia and Broncho-pneumonia. Morgan Pure is very often useful where the indicated remedy fails in asthma and is closely related to Natrum Sulph in asthma. Bronchitis every winter. Tendency to pneumonia. Never been well since pneumonia.

Suffocative attacks. Dyspnoea. Dry, tickling cough, loose cough.

Extremities

Numbness, tingling and neuritis. Diabetic neuropathy. Swelling of limbs and poor grip.

Cracked heels. Offensive foot sweat. Chilblains.

Varicose veins and ulcers.

Sleep and dreams

Insomnia if there is any light where they sleep - they must have everything dark around them and they are generally averse to bright light which also aggravates eye conditions and headaches, making them restless and irritable. Easily disturbed sleep.

Skin

Morgan Pure is the most important skin remedy- many symptoms in all areas and of all types including herpes, boils, fissures, eczema, impetigo, acne, dermatitis, prickly heat and erysipelas. Eruptions of all types but most frequently raw and discharging. Severe itching. It is also a singularly effective remedy for eczema during teething. The skin is dry and cracks particularly on the face, around the mouth and on the cheeks.

I had one young female patient with a face that looked like a dried-up reservoir and she needed Morgan and Psorinum to complete a cure that was begun by Natrum Mur.

There is intolerable itching (much worse than Mezereum or Fagopyrum) and great heat in skin complaints. Cannot tolerate wool next to skin. Itching sometimes diminishes when wearing silk.

General Modalities

Morgan Pure is worse for both fat and eggs. It may also crave or be averse. They can either crave or hate but whichever, if they crave it, it still makes them worse. It's not so bad if they are averse to them because they tend not to consume them but if they crave then that does produce a problem.

They are generally aggravated by storms and stormy atmospheres but they may also be affected by close atmospheres and very humid weather. They are worse at night and on rising in the morning.

Related remedies

Alumina	Baryta-carb.	Calcarea Carb.
Calcarea Sulph.	Carbo Veg.	Digitalis
Graphites	Kali Carb.	Magnesium Carb.
Natrum Carb.	Petroleum	Sepia
Sulphur		

Proteus

The keynote is **suddenness**.

The most common thing that people remember about Proteus is brain storm- fits of temper. If one thinks of Nux Vomica on a bad day then one could be thinking of a mild Proteus tantrum. These patients throw things harder and more often. They are easily irritated and averse to company, whilst being unable to bear difficulties, confrontations or contradictions.

I remember a colleague who gave Proteus to a patient, and two days later the patient was arrested for attacking his wife with a knife. Two years later he skipped with the financial assets of his business and left his partner in the lurch. He was not a nice individual and I think he summed up Proteus quite well. He was given the remedy for his headaches which did go away. It did work to that extent - I am not sure if he was violent beforehand, as he was not my patient, but I feel sure he must have been.

Proteus loses control - I think you would say with Proteus that their overall level of control is minimal. It doesn't require much to tip them over the edge. I remember going into a car park and I was ten yards behind the car in front because we were queuing - you go up these ramps and I waited at the bottom of the ramp because there was not a space clear at the top and the chap behind me wound down his window and gave me an extreme mouthful of abuse for not parking halfway up the ramp in the queue. I just ignored him and then he went to get out of the car to get at me. Happily, a space then appeared so I went up the ramp and he got back in the car. Very definitely capable of road rage - these are not nice people, and very confrontational.

As a corollary to their lack of control is a need to be, or appear to be, in control. Unfortunately for them this is very often a difficult thing to achieve, especially in these times of high stress in the world today and their lack of control of a situation often leads them to take actions as if they were in control. One way of pretending to themselves is to upgrade their I-phone, take a new lover or buy a new sports car, even if already deep in debt!

They are destructive and violent, prone to throw things, to kick and fight. They have tantrums as if they were a child.
As a personality, they tend to be unyielding, stubborn and unable to see someone else's point of view. They have fixed ideas usually relating to their own abilities and importance. You might even call it a delusion of their own importance. As well as that they can also lack self-confidence which also leads them to be domineering and aggressive, as a cover for their perceived inadequacy. They lie to exaggerate their own importance, and may even believe their tall tales.

They hate being contradicted and can be offended easily and are naturally quarrelsome. They have fears of open spaces, of the dark and of something unknown, but bad, being about to happen. Fear of losing his mind.
Proteus may be gloomy and melancholy, even appear to wallow in the emotion. They think they want to die but have no intention of committing suicide. They weep, moan and complain about their lot to others. They feel disrespected and that makes them angry. They find themselves unable to handle stress or questioning and again their refuge is usually anger.

Tendency to hysteria when he lets go of what controls he does have. He tends to keep himself to himself but likes to be respected from a distance. He is not a social creature since he considers most people to be not worth the trouble. They are mentally sharp or acerbic which compares with their physical tendency to be awkward or clumsy. This mental sharpness sometimes blunts, leaving them with mistakes in speaking and thinking., forgetting words and general mental confusion. Brain fag is the other end of the scale from brain storm.

In physical complaints and therapeutics, you are looking at complaints that come on suddenly and are spasmodic so you are looking at convulsions, cramps, epilepsy, and intermittent claudication, and anything which has suddenness about its onset. There also seems to be an element of the last straw about Proteus. These are people who cope with stress for a long time and then some little thing just tips them over the edge.

Proteus principally affects the nervous system. They also have a very high metabolic rate - you don't see many fat Proteans. These are the people who wake up at 2am and go downstairs and raid the fridge - eat a meal and go back upstairs to sleep again. Then have a full cooked breakfast the next morning. They use it up - they eat phenomenal amounts of food but are also known to have a lot of food fads, so they can be averse to almost anything although most commonly they are averse to greens and beans. So, if its salad they don't want it, and if it's a pulse they don't want it and they are not very good with onions and garlic either. There is usually a strong reaction, good or bad, to eggs in all forms. They may crave or be averse, but the reaction remains strong as is expected for someone with a tendency to allergies.

The trouble with the sudden onset part of their reactions, unlike your phosphorus where you get the thunderstorm and the sky clears quickly, with Proteus, it lingers on for days, so you get the sudden storm, but it doesn't abate. So it's like a volcanic explosion rather than a thunderstorm. I reckon the best thing to do with a Proteus when they do that is to feed them. They usually stop to eat – it's tiring having a tantrum so if they lose their temper, the best thing you can do is to put some food in front of them. They are prone to dependency on social drugs, especially alcohol, despite reacting easily and unpleasantly to overindulgence with hangovers and digestive upsets.

Generalities

Convulsions. Cramps and spasms. Allergies.
Neurasthenia. Neuritis. Slow recovery.

Head

The headaches are like Glonoine - sudden explosions in the brain with burning pains in the eyes. Headaches, if they don't come on suddenly tend to be associated with heavy forehead, worse mornings and with blurred vision. Pressing pains in head.

General frontal headache which debilitates but also makes him more irritable than ever, worse in the morning after rising. Head pain so bad that he hits his head to provide distraction.

Headaches increase before period.

Headaches associated with digestive upsets. Digestive migraines.

Alopecia in both sexes. Vertigo as if falling forwards, with coloured lights in vision. Vertigo whilst travelling.

Ears

Burning pains. As if swollen inside. Meniere's disease.

Eyes

They have photophobia and photosensitivity and generally tired and painful eyes. Burning or stitching pains make him press the eyes to relieve. Vision may be variable as he tires.

Nose

The nose is often blocked indoors. Post nasal discharge difficult to shift, feels glutinous.

Chronic rhinitis.

Mouth and Voice

There are cracks in the lips, especially in the corners. Salty taste. Prone to mouth ulcers. Furred tongue. Stammering in the child and the elderly.

Face

Dryness of lips. Cracks in the corners of the mouth. Herpes on lips. Acne especially on the lower jawline and chin.

Throat

A relaxed throat, or sometimes the opposite – a tight throat, makes speech difficult which adds to their temper and frustration. They are prone to acute pharyngitis. Dry throat with anxiety.

Chest and Heart

They have rattling mucous in the chest and there is bronchitis in the elderly.

Angina, coronary heart disease and cardiac pains generally. Palpitations from anxiety, stress or any strong emotion. Heavy weight in the chest.

Back

Copious sweat in axillae which drips down the arms. Boils in axillae.

Unspecific back aches. Numbness in the back. Poor nerve conductivity.

Respiration and lungs

Mucosal cough which is hard and tight. It sounds dry but eventually produces a little mucous.

Abdomen
Distention with flatus
Stomach and digestion
Acidity/heartburn/sourness.
Duodenal or gastric ulcers with associated pains and hunger pangs.
Flatulent distention. Flatus expelled up and down.
Pain when hungry but not relieved by eating. Emptiness which causes pain, not relieved by eating.
Nausea and head pains after eating. Vomiting after eating.
Aversion to dairy products and eggs but also may crave eggs. Aversion to salad and green vegetables, onions and chocolate.
Craves fats and sweets. Craving or aversion to butter.
Averse to chocolate, beef, pork, eggs and all raw food.
Loves rich food which aggravates.
Female
Leucorrhoea acrid, brownish and blood streaked. Worse before menses.
Leucorrhoea thick, white clotted, worse between menses.
Vaginitis, pruritis. Boils.
Menses of long duration, up to seven days with many fibrous clots.
Male
Unhealthy desire for sex. Violent sexual activity.
Incomplete erections.
Rectum and Stool
Like Nux Vomica, they have reverse peristalsis and rectal spasms. Blocked sensation in rectum.
Alternation of constipation and diarrhoea. Stress or excitement causes diarrhoea.
Soft, adhesive stools after rising from bed. Stools discoloured yellow.
Colitis pains sharp and stabbing.

Kidneys and Urinary

Cystitis associated with consuming food to which he is sensitive.

Burning pains in the urethra during urination.

Cloudy urine or with white sediment.

Pains in kidney described in colourful terms and as violent.

Pyelitis. Pyelonephritis.

Sleep and dreams

Their dreams are violent and filled with images of death, destruction and murder. Dreams of the dead and dying. Dreams of people he used to know.

Extremities

Numbness of hands or feet, associated also with burning sensations. They are also prone to cold and painful extremities < cold weather. Raynaud's syndrome.

Contracted tendons including Dupuytrens contracture

Intermittent claudication forces him to stop walking.

Phlebitis.

Sciatica

Cramps especially on exercise and in those who use their hands a lot like writers and musicians.

The remedy has done well for me, in several cases of RSI - where I have not given Proteus because they had RSI but the symptoms seems to have disappeared without recurrence after they have had Proteus.

Skin

They are prone to comedones, herpes, erythema, pruritis, cracks, fissures, peeling skin and genital boils, although there is nothing individualising about the skin symptoms. Herpetic eruptions at muco-cutaneous margins.

General Modalities

>After adjusting to moving around, or one hour after rising. Stretching. Eating. Lying down.

Feels better after drinking alcohol which later aggravates symptoms.
< Drinking alcohol. Exertion. Winter cold. Stormy weather. Night. Fats, garlic and rich food.

Related remedies

Apis	Cuprum	Coca
Ignatia	Nux Vomica	Strychnine

There follows an account of the Proteus proving the British School of Homoeopathy undertook in 2003 organised by Deborah Schofield and Lisa Mansell and supervised by Anthony Bickley

The proving started in January 2003 and concluded in May. 11 people took the substance - 10 women and 1 man. The majority of provers' symptoms stopped within 4-8 weeks. The provers selected their own proving potency by choosing from a range of numbered bottles, which resulted in 5 provers taking a 30c, 3 taking 1M and 3 taking 200c. No one selected placebo.

Methodology:

- 1 dose to be taken on the Sunday of the college weekend (Day 0)
- On Day 2, if - after consultation with the supervisor - it was felt that no
  symptoms had been experienced by the prover - a second dose was taken.
- If, after a further 5 days, no symptoms had been experienced, then a third and final dose would be taken. In the event however, no prover needed to take a third dose.

Proteus is a nosode, a potentised remedy made from a bacterium found in the gut.
Identified as a potential remedy by Edward Bach (of flower essences fame) and studied by Dr John Paterson who put together a clinical picture.
We chose Proteus to prove because it had not had a Hahnemannian proving. The clinical symptom picture we already had was compiled by studying sick people rather than a proving in which we study the effect on healthy people. It had a "masculine" picture which we felt might expand with predominantly female proving participants, and we were keen to use a substance likely to have a broad susceptibility which Proteus fulfilled as it is capable of living in the bowel of a large percentage of the population.

One of the most satisfying parts of this proving was the fact that symptoms produced by provers almost completely reconfirmed the existing picture and we also obtained some very striking new symptoms. It brought out extensive and valuable symptoms of which a summary follows.

Confirmation of existing symptoms:
Mental symptoms: anger, brainstorm, violent temper, nerve strain, fear of opinion of others, easily offended, vivid dreams of death, war. Aversion to company,
Physical symptoms: circulatory disorders, eggs - strong desire, spasms and cramps, herpetic eruptions, meibomian cyst, headaches/migraines, acidity, heartburn, ulcers. Itching. Split nails. Leucorrhea. Wine agg. need to eat and < > eating.

New and expanded symptoms:

Anger was often based in issues around what was "deserved", and desires were expressed more directly and effectively because of this. Clumsiness, issues around pregnancy and female identity. Libido changes, breast symptoms - larger, sorer, lactation, thickening of breast tissue. Ovulation symptoms and breakthrough bleeding, amenorrhoea, dysmenorrhoea. Skin - old scars itching, crusting and re-erupting, nbws chicken pox, Delusions/SRPs - taller, older, stabbed in back, fishhooks in scalp, hair standing on end, SAI heartbeat in urethra, SAI blunt instrument being forced into brain, vision of old lady, Sensation, when speaking/singing that someone else was doing it through them.
The proving started in January 2003 and concluded in May. 11 people took the substance - 10 women and 1 man. The majority of provers' symptoms stopped within 4-8 weeks. The provers selected their own proving potency by choosing from a range of unlabelled bottles, which resulted in 5 provers taking a 30c, 3 taking 1M and 3 taking 200c. No one chose placebo although there were bottles containing placebo in the selection.

Methodology

When considering the methodology to use in the proving we looked at various options.
We looked at Jeremy Sher's methodology, which is to give up to 3 doses a day for 2 days. Our feeling was that we did not want to repeat the remedy so frequently before knowing whether or not a symptom picture had started to develop.
We also bore in mind the fact that we knew from the existing picture that Proteus was a fast acting remedy and would not need as big a "kick" as a more psoric remedy.

Our intention therefore was to choose a methodology that would afford the maximum possibility of getting a result, without repeating it too frequently. We wanted to "push it" without overdoing it.
We therefore decided on the following:

> 1 dose to be taken on the Sunday of the college weekend (Day 0)
> On Day 2, if – after consultation with the supervisor – it was felt that no symptoms had been experienced by the prover – a second dose was taken.
>
> The instructions were that if, after a further 5 days, no symptoms had been experienced, then a third and final dose would be taken. In the event however, no prover needed to take a third dose.

....

Before the Proving started, we also asked the Supervisor to make a note of what they considered to be the constitutional remedy of their prover. The reason for this was that when assessing the action of the proving substance, we felt it important to know whether, for example, 9 out of the 11 provers were constitutionally Natrum Mur, or whether the substance could be said to have been proved on a wide-ranging spectrum of constitutional types.

Triad Sessions

When the provers' symptoms had finished, the next stage was to conduct triad sessions. This involved meeting with each prover and their supervisor and going through the diaries together to clarify any queries or to try to expand some symptoms. Before the meeting, we asked the prover and supervisor to go through their diaries individually, each highlighting those symptoms each felt to be true symptoms of the proving. They then went through the diaries together and highlighted any discrepancies. We then went through the diaries together and drew up a list of any queries we had. At the triad meeting we then had the opportunity to discuss these with the prover and the supervisor.

It all sounds a bit "long-winded", but we found the information obtained by the process invaluable. It enabled us to draw out some symptoms which had perhaps not seemed significant to the prover and, on the other hand, to discount some symptoms which on reading the diaries had seemed important.

Having gone through all the proving diaries, we also had the opportunity during these triad sessions to ask provers questions around themes we had noticed appearing in other diaries. This too yielded valuable information with provers adding detail they had not included in the diaries.

Proteus the remedy – what is it?

In homoeopathy, it is a nosode, a potentised remedy made from a bacterium found in the gut.

Identified as a potential remedy by Edward Bach (of flower essences fame) and studied by Dr John Paterson who put together a clinical picture, Murphy also credits Seveus as conducting a detailed study. Proteus has not had a Hahnemannian-type proving until now. The clinical symptom picture we already had was compiled by studying sick people rather than a proving in which we stud the effect on healthy people.

PROTEUS the remedy – Why?

Before starting the Proving, we drew up a shortlist of remedies we thought would make interesting proving substances. In Proteus, we identified several factors that we thought were important and would make it a suitable choice:

- Despite having had 'studies' carried out, there had not, to date, been a Hahnemannian proving. There is not much information available on Proteus or any of the bowel nosodes for that matter, in the Materia Medica texts with references currently only in Vermeulen and Murphy, so it is difficult to develop a broad understanding of the remedy and its potential.

- The existing picture was very limited – it is a small remedy and currently appears in only 53 rubrics in Synthesis.7.

- The picture that did exist was that of a very masculine remedy – it is often compared with Nux Vomica. With Proteus, we felt it unlikely that it would be prescribed for a woman, unless therapeutically as a specific for a condition such as RSI or intermittent claudication. We knew that with the female/male ratio at the BSH being what it is, a high percentage of the provers would be women and it would provide the opportunity to see if there was an undiscovered female side to the remedy which would therefore expand and balance the existing picture.

- Of course, when doing a proving, you always hope to get some clear, interesting symptoms that are experienced by several provers.
  This seems to validate the proving. Obviously, although no one knows exactly what will happen when the substance has been taken, we wanted, when selecting a proving substance, to try to use something that had a

good chance of having a high susceptibility rate amongst the provers. Since Proteus is a bacterium found in the gut, there was a good chance of having a high number of provers being susceptible to it.

The Symptoms

We thought we would present the proving information to you by outlining the leading symptoms already identified by Vermeulen/Murphy/Paterson and our own expert, Anthony Bickley. Describe how those symptoms were re-confirmed by our provers and expand to give you some of the symptoms discovered in this proving. Where appropriate, we will give you the actual words of the Prover.

Mental/Emotional

Nux Vomica on a bad day = Proteus on a good day.
Several provers reported feeling in a Nux Vomica state. But in Proteus there is even more rage/anger/irritability - the word "brainstorm" is used to describe it. A lot of our provers certainly felt it - these are quotes:

- *Anger, which feels uncomfortable because I have not been angry for years.*

- *I have been cross, impatient and snappy. Snatched pen from a colleague.*

- *The things I want to say involve swearing and are very aggressive.*

- *Exceedingly bad tempered, very angry. Flipped over something I was furious about. Reaction was over the top.*

- *Had a customer who seemed to be trying to make me hit her.*

- *Need a discharge of anger. At any time feel I could blow my top.*

- *Feel sharp, but sort of irritable. I'm not taking crap from anybody sort of mood. Like Nux Vomica.*

This already known aspect of Proteus, caused us some concern as proving coordinators. We considered that some of our provers did have some Nux type aspects and were worried that the substance might make them literally blow up with anger. This didn't seem to happen, those provers often felt less angry than normal which might mean the Proteus was acting curatively in them. The people who did have the rage were those who were constitutionally more suppressed remedies, Proteus seemed to remove the block!
The language of the provers when describing physical symptoms reflected this state. They talked, for example, of Furious (energy), explosive (diarrhoea), violent (sneezing), angry (skin).

This very aggressive state has in the past been seen as totally negative. In our provers however, it was tempered by a positive aspect. Several provers felt able through this anger, to confront issues and communicate their desires for the first time. Even when anger was not involved, this was a theme – Provers felt that they should get what they deserved.

- *I expressed what I thought I deserved and desired and criticised others.*

- *I feel I just want to have a good time. I would like to be more selfish about it, but I am not a selfish person.*

- *I've been communicating my desires more effectively.*

- *I've been saying things more directly.*

- *Finally spoke up for what I wanted.*

- *Didn't feel guilty about coming back late from lunch – felt like I deserved it.*

The original picture has large ego, superiority and self-importance and there were elements of this recorded by our provers. They mentioned feeling aloof and detached and felt that others could not do things properly or as well as them. They felt apart from others.

- *No longer care about others. Own desires more important, want to take things for myself.*

- *Felt very frustrated at work – as if everyone was dong things wrongly, or too slowly.*

- *Felt distant and separated from others ….very tall.*

- *Felt separate and much taller than the others and older – as if I was their parent. Felt disconnected from them.*

This aspect leads rather nicely into some SRP symptoms that were experienced:
Delusions of being larger/taller.

- *I feel very tall and looking out of my bedroom window I thought "I'm on top of the world here. I seem to be higher than everywhere."*

- *I have the sensation of a cylinder on top of my head rising up.*

- *Felt sides of head were being lifted up like tiny fishing hooks, tiny pinpricks lifting up.*

This idea of fishhooks includes the theme of sharpness that cropped up several times in various guises. Provers felt sharp - one prover even had the sudden delusion that she had been stabbed in the back - not metaphorically, but actually. Another described a pain in the occiput as being a stabbing pain. Physically too, there were symptoms of sharp edges.

- *Stool painful again – feels like a sharp edge when passing.*

- *Sensation of hard edges in my stomach like hardback books in there. I can feel the edges when the squeezing starts.*

There were also dreams of stabbings. It was a feature of this proving that there were numerous dreams, many of which involved death, dying, murder – this type of dream is already in the picture.
The mental sharpness seems to have a strong polarity of awkwardness and clumsiness, both physically, where people tripped and dropped things, but also in expression:

- *Clumsy. Tripped twice walking and couldn't open the door.*

- *Fell downstairs and twisted left ankle.*

- *Fell over step on front door hurting right shin – just clumsy.*

- *Noticed I was making mistakes in writing – switching round 1st and 2nd letters of words. Writing bad. Couldn't spell, couldn't get the words, a load of scribble. Words don't look right.*

- *Mental confusion, inability to articulate, to find the right word, using wrong words. This to the point it was disturbing.*

- *Less able to communicate during proving. Mishear, misunderstand or misappropriate words. Totally out of control.*

Someone in a Proteus state is using up a huge amount of energy which needs replacing. Nearly all our provers felt hungry immediately after taking the substance, and several noted a huge increase in appetite during the proving, but not an increase in weight. A Proteus keynote is getting up in the middle of the night to eat and some provers experienced this. Others ate breakfast when they normally wouldn't, because they were ravenous. Some got up early so they could eat. One prover who had been a vegetarian for most of their life suddenly craved some sausages that were at the family's house. The craving went on for a couple of hours until they finally ate them.

Eggs - craving/aversion/aggravation - keynote of Proteus. Other provers were craving boiled eggs, egg and bacon etc.

- *Very hungry at 3.30. Look forward to going home to nibble – a severe need today of soft boiled eggs.*
- *Went to get egg sandwiches and bought 3. felt myself craving boiled egg sandwich this morning. Thinking about this when working instead of the work.*

Food and its effect on blood sugar was an important factor. Provers "had" to eat, were > or < for eating and one prover with diagnosed hypoglycaemia felt the substance had acted curatively for the duration of the proving.
Alcohol: Several provers had severe cravings for beer, wine, spirits, but they paid for it. Alcohol effects and hangover symptoms were out of proportion to the amount of alcohol drunk. This was a symptom experienced by most of the provers.

Female

We mentioned earlier that one of the reasons for choosing Proteus as the proving substance was because the known picture was a very masculine one and we felt that it would be interesting to see if the remedy could be found to have a more female side. Something that has been particularly interesting for us is that the remedy has a strong hormonal connection and can produce very striking symptoms relating to The Feminine.
With the anger, we saw that there was a very confrontational aspect and this sense of confrontation can also be seen here. Proteus seems to make women confront their femininity - both on the emotional and on the physical levels. These are not subtle, mild symptoms, but symptoms that make you take notice of them - they cannot be ignored. There is a constant reminder of the feminine.
On the physical side, this gave symptoms such as protracted, more noticeable ovulation, ovulation pain, strong ovulation symptoms such as spotting and increased leucorrhoea. Menses were heavy, clotted and flooding or in contrast, one prover's periods stopped for the entire duration of the proving.

On the emotional side, there were some very powerful experiences relating to "the feminine". One prover, for example, found herself confronting the issue of wanting to have children - obviously the most fundamental aspect of The Feminine. In a relationship where she wanted children but her partner did not, she found herself thinking about it all over again, having thought that the issue had been resolved. She described experiencing during the proving feelings of "inadequacy as a woman", "a discomfort with being female". She described having difficulty in "coming to terms with the feminine as a part of me because I don't have children. I married someone who didn't and I squashed my desire down. These feelings led to her wanting to withdraw from her partner, not wanting to be touched. This same prover also described getting angry "in an hysterical, womanly way".

Another prover who said that she had been thinking more about pregnancy and feeling "gushy" about it during the proving found herself experiencing breakthrough bleeding at mid-cycle although she was on the pill - as if her body was drawing her attention to the possibility or the need to have a child and not wanting to have that suppressed by the pill.
In both these examples, the provers appear to have experienced a strong reaction against the suppression of The Feminine - in the first prover, against the suppression of her natural feminine instinct to have children and in the second, against the physical suppression through the use of the pill.
Proteus had a marked effect on libido. Some experienced a much higher libido than usual. They described wanting sex all the time, thinking about it all day. They referred to having a "heightened desire" and being "more passionate" and "more playful". The polarity to this was a reduced libido with some provers not wanting sex at all or describing feeling unsexual. Some took longer than usual to reach orgasm or were unable to reach orgasm at all. For some provers, this lack of desire could be put down to the physical symptoms.
Sex felt uncomfortable because of symptoms such as vaginal soreness and itching or the sensation of the vagina being bruised.

The sexual theme continued in the dreams. There were several sexual and erotic dreams and interestingly, provers made the comment that it felt strange to have such strongly sexual dreams when physically they felt unsexual.
The provers themselves often likened their symptoms to those of puberty, pregnancy, lactation and PMT. There was nausea on waking - similar to morning sickness and also some urinary symptoms which brought pregnancy to mind. Some provers - and also supervisors - experienced the "let down" reflex sensation of breastfeeding. Interesting, when this was mentioned at Bath on the day we revealed our findings, several people came up to us afterwards and said they had experienced this sensation during the proving - even though they were not directly involved.

The theme of pregnancy and motherhood also extended through to the sub-conscious, with several provers having dreams of babies - one dreamt that she offered to breastfeed a very large baby and another dreamt of being woken by a baby crying next door.

- *Bladder feels weak. Strong feeling I could be incontinent.*

- *Felt I couldn't hold urine in. Urethra felt weak.*

- *Breasts feel bigger and sorer than normal before a period.*

- *Breasts feel as if they could breastfeed triplets – huge, and also that prickly, tingly feeling when breastfeeding.*

- *Nauseous – feels like morning sickness.*

- *Wake at 4.00 with hormonal thing – haven't had this for a long time.*

- *Seriously would love to put a baby to the breast.*

- *I have been thinking a lot more about pregnancy recently – more gushy.*

- *I look 5 months pregnant.*

- *Sudden striking pain – this is a symptom I've only ever had when pregnant.*

Headaches

Migraines - especially those which are blinding and sudden - were already in the picture and this was certainly confirmed by the proving. Some provers reported experiencing more headaches than usual. A positive result was that for some provers, migraines were a cured symptom, reporting that they did not experience headaches in situations that would normally have provoked them.

- *Not getting migraines as I would normally*

- *migraine came on much quicker than normal*

- *migraine headache with nausea, numbness and tingling*

Circulatory Disorders

Proteus is used therapeutically as a specific for Raynaud's Syndrome, Repetitive Strain Injury, Intermittent Claudication. Our results confirmed these symptoms. There were icy and numb hands and feet, writer's cramp and inability to type, cramps in calves < cycling and running.

- *couldn't continue to run legs feel almost too heavy to lift*

- *Feeling cold in extremities, I can't seem to get warm even when had a hot bath*

- *Had to stop entering data on computer because hand hurt so much from repetition*

Gut

Proteus is an explosive remedy and as you might expect, this carried through to the gut. A lot of air was emitted in both directions. There was spasm and pain in the stomach and one prover had a return of symptoms from an ulcer - duodenal ulcers are already in the Proteus picture.
Several provers also reported nausea and acidity and an increased sensitivity to what they ate.

- *Explosive diarrhoea after coffee*
- *General unease due to the possibility of explosive stools*
- *Woke up feeling slightly sick, like too much acid in the stomach, very loud burping, lots of air.*

Skin

Herpetic eruptions were already in the existing picture. Several provers developed cold sores or felt as if one were developing. This was also one of the cured symptoms of the proving. Very interestingly, one prover who had been seriously ill with chickenpox in recent years and had "Never been well since" had the experience of their old chickenpox scars itching and spots then forming again in those places. At the end of the proving they felt that they had regained their "Pre-chickenpox state".
The following are quotes taken from this provers experience through the proving

Prover 20211
Day 6: Old chicken pox scars itching
Day 8: So many spots am like a dalmation, all chicken pox scars have erupted and there are others on chin and nose.
Day 9: Old chicken pox scar eruptions till there raised on the outside.
Day 12: Large painful chicken pox scars on the back of the next < RS
Day 24: State of health has returned to pre-chicken pox state 6 years ago.
Day 24: Old friends have come and sought me out, including those I haven't seen since before I had chicken pox.

Provers experienced severe itching – in all parts of the body, but particularly on, in and around the genitals.

- *Genital itching over penis and testicles particularly base of abdomen to base of penis.*

- *Intense all over and deep inside itching, vaginal itchiness*

Notably, in view of the "re-activation" of the chickenpox scars, other provers noticed changes in surgical scars for example caesarean and episiotomy scars and scars from the removal of varicose veins.

- *Scars from varicose vein operation were itchy and went crusty.*

- *Episiotomy scar itchy.*

Boils, (slowly developing) also formed part of the old picture and this symptom was borne out by the proving.

THEMES

To summarise, from what we have seen so far, various themes stand out in Proteus:

Confrontation:
The mental picture showed this in the anger manifested by the provers. Also in the more positive aspect of people confronting issues and feeling they should get what they deserved. Proteus also seemed to stimulate in provers the energy, will, desire or need to confront issues from the past that they had, for whatever reason, suppressed. The physical symptoms were also confrontational – explosive, "in your face" symptoms that made people sit up and take notice of them.

Rigidity:
On the mental/emotional side, rigidity and inflexibility can be seen in the selfishness that was experienced by some provers, believing their own desires to be more important than those of others. Also, provers seemed very unyielding in their attitude.
They quickly became very impatient with other people. Physically, this theme continues with the sensation of sharpness and hardness, the RSI symptoms, cramping and Raynaud's.

Communication:
Linked perhaps to the confrontational aspect is the sense that the remedy can open up lines of communication. Provers described being able to say things more directly, to communicate their desires more effectively, to speak up for what they wanted. When we were going through the diaries, we noticed that several provers had felt moved to renew contact with people from their past with whom they had lost touch. This seemed significant enough to ask other provers about it during the triad sessions and we found that this had happened to others as well. Also - slightly spookily - a significant enough number of provers for it to be more than a coincidence found that during the proving, people from their past renewed contact with them after a long time.

Other SRPs
SAI as if ice had been applied to vagina and inner thighs
sensation of a heartbeat in the urethra
SAI blunt instrument was being forced gently but rhythmically up into brain.
SAI and actual appearance of hair follicles standing on end like a hedgehog.
Vision of old lady hovering above
Delusion that although they were speaking/singing it was someone else doing so, saying things they wouldn't say, or in a different way to they would say it, or hymns!

Related remedies.

In addition to those remedies already noted in Murphy: Apis, Cuprum, Nat. Mur
We would also suggest connections with
Nux Vomica
Sepia
Lac Humanum – two provers were independently prescribed this remedy after the proving
Folliculinum
Silica
Sycotic Co

DREAMS

PROVER NO. 1

DAY 3

I have had dreams of dogs twice since taking remedy. It's a good feeling toward them – I'm quite sure the dogs are the ones I used to have. Also I specifically remember fleas in my dream. This morning I noticed black specks on my shirt and thought of fleas – this is what reminded me of that aspect of that dream.

DAY 4

Dreamt of Dev (from television programme "Coronation Street") and "comfort" because I was lost in a casino-type place for a while – then found him. Discussed sleeping together. He didn't want to use a condom because it "tickled". I did not want to do without.

Also dreamt that I was pulling a hair out of my mole on my chin and ended up pulling a rock-like feature out (to the point where it was distorting my mouth). I regretted this, but it wouldn't fit back!

Great Dane present in dream as well.

DAY 6

Dreamt that I had been in a bad cycling accident and had been "put back together" but in a strange way. Someone reminded me that my organs etc were not where they are normally. i.e. I had a can of lager in my shoulder and a pack of cigarettes in my arm (amongst my real organs) which were displaced.
This showed up in an x-ray. I also had photos in there as well - including pix of my dog and some pix of my youth etc. Something had obviously happened to my family as I felt sad and happy looking at these memories. A lot of people from work were there - most of them watching a presentation. I was watching them instead.

DAY 8

This one centred around a race/fun run. I did it with a few people including my boyfriend. Did it in about 1 hour 20, but to get our times written we had to wait in a queue. This was taking a long time, so I left the queue. I saw no point - the time would show up as a long time. I was also very bored in listening to what people talked about. I constantly needed distraction i.e. a girl did a quiz to help us pass time. The other thing was that I had a little bag of fish which included very small ones - some alive, some dead, which we were meant to eat. I thought this very strange. I didn't know this place very well.

DAY 12

Background: The area we are housesitting in is near one of the roughest parts in Oxford. I first found out how close we were yesterday, although the place at hand is very nice. Anyway, in dream, we were a bunch of people at friend's house in the same area – everyone else was in a room and I was listening/watching music on a player. I went for a walk and someone from the area told me that she'd heard a rape happening the other day. Then, for some reason, I was with another friend and walking back to that house, we saw two cops entering another house. There had been a murder/attack. I saw a sharp gardening tool on the pavement and told the lady who was in the house with the cops. When went back to our friends, my dumb friend handed me over the instrument. I was very upset. I had touched it, so had she. Worried about housesitting thereafter.

DAY 19

Was in a tent-like place with my boyfriend where there were others as well. We'd just walked in and for some reason, I was naked. The guy in front, who had very long whitish/blond hair just looked at my breast and said that he'd always dreamt of hooters like that (and his girlfriend was just beside him). I told him to fuck off. Then we started throwing insults back and forth. I'm not sure what I did to him first, but the next thing, we were wrestling and hurting each other. It was only when he started digging with his nail on my right calf a long time (and it was hurting a long time) and it started bleeding, that he stopped and left. The blood was normal at first, then went muddy/oily/watery brown after he let go. He left before realising the amount of blood. Woke up and felt pain in right calf.

DAY 27

Dreamt about work. I had applied for another job in the same company. I had been accepted and was due to start. All of a sudden, I realised I was happy where I was and declined the job. I felt very good and proud to be loyal to it. I think it was also quite courageous to quit just before starting as well – but it was what I wanted.

DAY 29

Had a dream about the high school reunion I will be attending in May. Arrived expecting to see loads of people I knew although not many people were there yet. I was really excited when I saw this girl I knew with her Dad, twin sister and 3 kids. She was eating very green olives (many in a bowl. She didn't speak to me so her Dad said they weren't here to socialize – they wanted a signature from the principal and that was it. She never looked up. (NB This is based on some truth – she never wants to do anything with this school again).

DAY 32

Dreamt of sex last night.

DAY 41

My Mum was generally a kind of medium for ghosts in that she could help people understand/communicate with them. She told me there was something one had to tell me (although she knew what this was). I hadn't been in this situation before, but felt quite comfortable with it. At one point this awful screeching sound was heard. I knew it was the ghost and I opened the door. The scary/old figure came up to me, arms drawn out, and pressed into my eyeballs with much force. It hurt very much. My Mum told it to stop and it did, but not before doing it once more. It was not a predicament about a disease, but basically a way of realising I was lucky my eyes worked. We had to tell the ghost to leave me alone and let me have them until I wasn't meant to anymore. I woke up right on time before my alarm – it was quite an unnerving dream.

DAY 45

Dreamt of playing football for Oxford United (!). My foot seemed not to remember how to strike a ball – ended up going towards own side, but then person behind me scored (for our team) – hooray!

PROVER NO. 2

DAY 3

Dream: Had text from my husband. "To my darling wife – this may be the last time you ever hear from me". I could picture him in a cave – he'd gone caving/potholing and he was stuck – danger. I was very upset.

DAY 6

Very erotic dream – being kissed. Strange, as I feel completely unsexual at present.

PROVER NO. 3

DAY 1

Dreamt I was with my brother and some friends. We were on London Underground. We were lost or rather didn't know where we were. We asked a guard who was up some stairs at the station and he told us a place we had never heard of. Next we went down some stairs and were in the bottom of a multi-storey car park. A black limousine drove past and stopped. It had the back cut out like a pick-up truck and there were 5 objects wriggling around under a bright flowered duvet cover. It was mainly red, everything else was black/grey and dreary. The duvet was lifted and it was 5 refugee children all under 6 with huge eyes. They were dirty. A wealthy Indian woman got out of the car. She had lots of gold jewellery on. I woke up.

DAY 2

Very vivid dream. Was shoe shopping in department store. It was Debenhams. I was present in dream. I could see me. I wanted these shoes and I'd been waiting 25 minutes for service. People were milling about and when an assistant came out she went to serve a guy who had just arrived. I very politely told her that there had been others waiting and she laughed a demonic laugh and told me to "sit down you bitch". When I said "don't talk like that" she stabbed me in the mouth with a knitting needle until blood was drawn. Bizarrely the stabbing came from inside cheek out. It was only my left cheek. Then I woke up. This dream happened 5-6am - ish. Woke feeling very irritable and snapped at the kids.

DAY 3

Dreamt again last night - can't remember it well....at friend's house but it wasn't her house cos this one was posh and well-furnished - my friends isn't. Didn't feel well in my dream and my friend put me to sleep in her son's bed. She woke me up after an hour and said she didn't think I'd want to sleep longer.
Suddenly I was watching a police drama on tv and a colleague was sitting next to me like an old man with a blanket over his legs. He was eating a KitKat - biting chunks from the side. It was very messy. He said hello to me and we chatted and I then realised he was also on tv, as a detective, at the same time as he was talking to me. Struck by the fact that he had a beard. I woke up.

DAY 4

Dreamt several times. I was with my brother and his mates and we went for a walk and turned a corner and met a flood. We couldn't pass this flowed into me being lost with friends in a large college building. We turned the corner and walked into a homoeopathy lecture being run by a well-known homoeopath. It became her college and we didn't want it to be seen as if we were saying we weren't. we tried to run and hid in a lift shaft. Turned another corner and this homoeopath was there. She asked us to look after her daughter. We went shopping and then I woke up. Felt very anxious on waking.

DAY 6

Dreamt of knives and studying. Can't remember any more except it wasn't a bad dream.

DAY 9

Dreamt of an old college tutor. It was to do with me studying for my A Levels. All a bit confused.

DAY 12

Dreamt again, another scenario. I was on the beach with yr 4 students and we were hunting fish in rock pols with hunting knives. It was not for fun for for food, but was still enjoyable. Then switched to being in a classroom. I was suddenly on the phone to a student's husband and he was demanding to talk to her. Told him she wasn't there and he said "you told me that before you bitch and you were wrong, I'll sort you out".

When the student came into the room and I told her, her husband was still on the phone and it was a menacing call. The dream ended here.

DAY 13

Very weird dream. We were in a large house with lots of little rooms and it was a "proving house". I saw 2 colleagues and apologised for being irritable and tetchy. One said he understood why I'd been a cow but his partner didn't. she said everybody was having trouble with how I'd been and suddenly I was in the middle of a circle of people and was crying. They were proving people, I was saying I was sorry and I ran away. They didn't believe me. I ran into a little room and saw my toddler son playing. I couldn't cope with him so ran away. I felt guilty I saw more provers and I tried to explain that I was on a proving too, but they wouldn't believe me. I woke up.

DAY 15

Nightmare, had to get out of bed to open window. Unusual. Couldn't remember nightmare.

PROVER NO. 4

DAY 6

Dreamt was at a homoeopathic college having an interview. Talking with the other students I felt like I didn't know enough (some specific things around this happened which I can't remember). Then I saw the head of the college who was a skinny man with huge, bright red hair, sticking straight out in large curly frizz. Looked like Side Show Bob off the Simpsons. He was just starting to tell me something about provings when the dream was interrupted by my son waking up at about 4.00am.

Interpretation: left over feelings from the weekend. Lack of confidence - I'm not learning enough, I'm not knowledgeable enough. The new college means I'm desiring more - the exact issues from Sunday.

PROVER NO. 7

DAY 2

Very intense dream, which I can even remember (this does not happen often): I am in a hotel in the country with a man I love, but he is dangerous and might kill other people. So I decide to kill him before he can do any harm. He is in the bathroom shaving. I come in with a knife hidden in my hand to kill him, but on the way I decide I cannot do it and kiss him instead. He discovers the knife in my hand and realises what I was planning to do, but can't. He turns the blade in the palm of my hand so deep that the cut should always remind me of him. There is a lot of blood. I flee and realize that I have to get help from the village but the wooden stairs to get out of the hotel were freshly painted and the owner of the hotel warns me that everything is very slippery, so I glide down these stairs (more like a ladder) with hands and feet, but I make it and wake up by my alarm clock.

DAY 3

Dreamt about living on a blanket fixed over 4 high poles, very free feeling, everybody else lived like this as well.

DAY 14

Had a nightmare: I took an old client of mine out for lunch and picked him up at home. To get to his garage and his car we had to climb a very steep iron staircase which became a narrow bridge across a road. My client was really struggling to make it up there. I asked him why he did not move to a more accessible place, but he claimed that the exercise was good for him.
On top of the bridge, he suddenly slipped between the bottom and the banister and fell onto the street. To me it looked like suicide, but I could not be sure. I ran to the street and there he lay with many other dead people and they all looked like puppets. They had shrunk and especially their heads were very small and painted a bit like clowns.

I was shocked to see my client like this. I could not recognize him anymore. Then I bumped into an old friend of mine who told me she had come especially to have a look at these dead people as there is a new method to prepare the bodies after death to make them look so beautiful - and yes, aren't they beautiful. She was planning to commit suicide herself but wanted to make sure, that she would be beautiful like this. Then I woke up and the image of this strange, painted, shrunken head was still with me in the morning.

DAY 21

Dream: Walk down a village street in the deep snow, dressed in bathrobe and slippers in the middle of the night to bring back a hoover I had borrowed. Suddenly a car comes along and stops just as I reach the house. People get out of the car. I am very scared and hide behind the house, then wake up and the fear of being hurt stays with me for a while.

DAY 26

Swissair launched two new planes and were filling them up with people. I was in one of them. I saw the other plane doing a loop just after take-off and falling on its back on the ground exploding. I was not so much frightened, but concerned that my family would not know in which plane I was.

DAY 33

Dream I am woken up by a baby crying next door. I realise I had completely forgotten I had a child and had not fed it all day. Felt really bad I forgot about that, then I realise I had a dog as well which I had also not fed and neglected. Woke up feeling really bad.

PROVER NO. 8

DAY 1

Dream where I was asleep under the sea but at the shore line, lying on my stomach. As I began to wake, I let my body float towards the shore until my belly touched the stones of the beach and I could sit up out of the water. My husband was sitting there on the beach as were a few other people to the left. The beach was made of rough reddish stones and the tide was coming in fast towards the cliff behind. I said: "Have I been asleep?" and husband answered "Yes, for ages". I remember thinking "Great, I feel refreshed. It's done me good to have this sleep."

DAY 2

Somewhere between 7.15am and 7.45am – sexual dream. Having sex with husband and meanwhile a black man and black woman are having sex on a big movie screen behind us. Then in the middle of this, husband stops having sex with me in order to eat a small red tomato which he has in a jar by the bed. He is then walking around and I am very frustrated (!).

DAY 3

I am in a snake pit with thousands of different types of snakes squirming around. So many, I am literally having to stand on some of them. I am not bitten. I seize one snake – a smaller sized one that is rusty red coloured and creamy white. He seems to be the most vicious and deadly.

My thought is that if I can control him then I will not be harmed. I hold him in my right hand, just down from his neck area, so although he tries, if he turns his head back to try to bite me he cannot reach. So I hold him out like this as a weapon against all the other snakes and indeed against anything else which may wish to hurt me.

Gradually I feel as if we are at one (although I wouldn't completely trust him – he is so vicious and deadly. He bites other snakes and they die immediately. Then a giant lizard and other small lizards are there. I am terrified by this huge lizard, but my snake easily kills it. I am not sure as to the ending, but I'm sure I end up putting the snake into a swimming pool which is inside a house. There are lots of other creatures (I can't think what sort in the pool).

(NB Bear in mind, my Mum is about to move house tomorrow in real life and I am helping her).
I am in a furniture van – a huge lorry – which alternates in terms of the driver between my ex-husband and my father (both incompetent men). We are driving all over everywhere including the village I used to live in in Cornwall. Sometimes the drive is treacherous eg reversing down an almost vertical wall. I am angry and frustrated and tearful. We arrive at my Mum's new place. It is late in the evening, everything is in a mess and I am upset.

DAY 4

Dreams came thick and fast, but difficult to remember. One about a big café (like Boston T Party) in which they served delicious afternoon teas with currant cakes.(!).

DAY 6

Frustration at husband who is talking to another guy about the kids and then pretending he is on the proving! Then a stroppy teenage girl says she has always been in love with my husband. (I am by now well pissed off!). she starts acting very madly still saying she wanted sex with my husband. Her mother announces that this girl is on speed.
Everyone (including my husband) thinks that this is an admirable excuse for her behaviour. Then he appears wrapped only in a towel. I say "how come you have just been with her and come back naked?" Then she appears in a towel. My husband says: "I have just made love to a girl on speed and I feel like I'm the only man in the world." I go into a crying, jealous, frenzy. Then I wake up whimpering

....

An epic dream. By this I mean it seemed to last ages – like watching a film. I can't remember enough detail to document it properly, but it starts in the past in a former generation. There is an old woman crawling on the floor and she eats some pieces of paper to get rid of what appears to be clues leading to a fortune of money. She is then killed by a black man. It then seems as we pass through time that this money is to pass in inheritance to a son. The dream is awash with different characters trying to get the money. At the end it is my mum, dad and me. There are lies being told about the money and about a piece of paper that will give the evidence as to who should have it. I trick them into giving me the piece of paper then screw it up and throw it onto the fire and say "Now no one can have it". There are a lot more unremembered details.

DAY 7

Long elaborate dreams not remembered well enough to write down. As if I have long epic dreams interspersed with snapshot quick fleeting dreams/images.

DAY 9

Highly sexual dream between 7am and 7.45am. No gory details – just a strong desire for sex.

....

Very angry and frustrated on arriving at my clinic with all my patients following me upstairs. Then husband still in clinic and won't leave. The room is a total mess. I am crying and frustrated and angry, but when I try to speak, my throat is constricted and I can hardly talk. Husband says, we'll have to sort you out (as if there's something wrong with me). The receptionist said: "I think you've had a stroke. Everyone else is laid back not minding, whilst I'm struggling and can't speak, with no one helping me.

....

Another frustrating dream: I was interviewed as a teacher and had to take a class in a school which I did ok. I then had to meet my interviewers who asked me to go and get them cups of tea and coffee. Given my circumstances, I dutifully go, but being desperate for a pee, I need to go before continuing my interview. Trying to juggle all these things I eventually find some toilets and try to avoid another woman's menstrual blood which I do get some on my hands. The dream dispersed, but again frustrating.

DAY 10

Another sexually orientated dream at some point. This seems peculiar given that in waking life with my exaggerated PMT state, sex is not an option!

DAY 11

I do have the same amount of dreams. Intense and small dreams, and I wake between each. I cannot remember enough detail to record except interestingly in one I offer to breastfeed a rather large baby.

DAY 13

Anger, tears and frustration when I am teaching a class and they do not like me or my methods. They are all being really horrid and I am trying to make myself heard and understood.

....

I am in a large 'sports hall' where loads of young people are being put through some army training. They have to work through a set sequence of almost dance like movements. There are 2 men leading them through this 'routine'. In this dream I am more like a 'guest teacher' and feel that (as opposed to the previous dream) well-known and respected. At one point, my left eye feels "gritty" and I wipe it with my finger and remove either a tiny orange ant or spider – I can't tell which it is.

DAY 16

Dream of visiting my Dad's unborn baby. I was talking to it.

DAY 18

I am dying of cancer with only 2 hours left to live and I am in a 'hospice'. Although I am dying I don't feel ill and I am preparing to die just as one might prepare to give birth. I am thinking about my death in a philosophical way. I go into a 'kitchen' area and notice how badly the walls are cracked and how badly it is kept. Then I think (or someone says) that when people just come here to die there is no point in keeping it any other way. I look at all the cups and think: a while ago someone drank out of these and now they are dead and gone and forgotten. How quickly life moves by. Soon I will be dead and my cup will remain for someone else to use – how quickly life passes through us. In my room all is white and bright. I think some people sit at one end but I can't see who they are. My husband sits by my bed. I am waiting to die – for it to be my turn. I feel I can see heaven. I see lots of beautifully coloured flowers (like sweet peas). I tell my husband. He says he can see them too. I tell him – no, you can only *imagine* them, I can *see* them.

(Day 19 – I tell husband about dream and feel tearful).

DAY 21

2 dreams:
Frustration and anger at work/with husband. I can't finish what I need to. Frustrated with husband who is not quick/efficient enough. He hangs phone up on me. (In real life we never row).

………………………………………………

I cannot describe this dream in detail. It was intense and packed full of symbols. For instance, a scarecrow type model made from black feathers. In a house at night trying to lock doors and windows to keep out 'the predator'.

………………………………………………………

Note: In general, in this proving my dreams have been intense, packed full of either detail or comprised of small mini-dreams – so much so that they make you feel almost exhausted on waking. Also, it has been hard to remember them in as much detail as I would like, but occasionally during the days a thought/image has occurred to me which I then associate with being part of a dream. I do dream very regularly and very intensely/profoundly at times. I am not sure therefore how much these dreams are different on the proving except to say I think I have had more than usual and more varied.

DAY 29

(NB The programme I had watched on TV was about Judgement Day/End of the World.).
At home with my husband and children we are aware it is the end of the world. There is a news programme on TV saying this, but the broadcast cannot continue. The sky outside is dark and clouds are rolling around moving quickly. The sky seems to be reeling with strange phenomenon. I am sitting with my family waiting for the 'final moment' which doesn't actually come.
It then moves on to me being out in a town somewhere. I observe almost like watching TV coverage, how the world will end. Even at one point it is as if watching the world from in space so one can see the outline of the countries on the globe. I am told that the first place to go will be a coastline area in France where all the wealthy go on holiday. Then slowly other places would be destroyed.
The way this was to happen was for a hot molten lava to come over the sea, onto the sea shore and spread across the land.
I am witness to this happening the first time. The red-hot lava comes in, - carried by the sea it spreads quickly. People are running away. Some are killed. Because of the nature of the coast, the lava is soon stopped in its flow.
Next time I am on the beach. I am shouting to people that this will happen again. I see the red-hot lava coming across the sea in the distance. Everyone starts to run as fast as possible away from the beach and into the town.

I run as fast as I can as the lava is spreading very quickly destroying everything in its path. I run through a tunnel and then reach a metal staircase. I climb up the stairs to avoid the lava. From this high point I can see the terror of it spreading across the town. I know that once it has run its course, it will cool down and turn black, then stop. This is does, just as it reaches the bottom of the staircase I'm standing on.

I felt this was a very powerful dream. I woke myself up from it and thought I must remember the details. When I went back to sleep, I dreamt the whole thing a second time.

DAY 30

Long epic dream about being in Ireland visiting a friend.

DAY 33

In the dream, someone says to me – There's no way of saying this Mrs X, but you have cancer in your bones, in your liver and in your spleen.

PROVER NO. 10

DAY 16

Dream of having 4 flat tyres.

DAY 37

Had a dream about 2 friends in their late 30's who were expecting a baby. I haven't seen them since the New Year so I know they have talked about children in the past. They got married 4 years ago but she was told she would probably not be able to have any. Must phone them to see how they are.

PROVER NO. 11

DAY 21

Dreamt last night. Can't recall what about, but it was a nightmare or I have the feeling it was.

PROVER NO 13

DAY 0

Lots of muddled dreams. Can't remember much, only that a lot of cheese was involved. Cheese seemed to keep cropping up. I had won some cheese and it was ½ eaten. I stole some cheese from someone too.

DAY 2

Dreams of old work place, of being at work.
Some Asians stopped me walking out of a shop. They wanted to check my bag, said I had stolen something. Feeling of indignation.
DAY 6

Muddled dreams, lots of them. No particular theme. I remember trying to find a caravan, somewhere to sleep, but it was all too small.

DAY 7

Dreamt boyfriend was shorter than I remembered him to be, a dwarf in fact. I couldn't remember him to be that small. He got some work on TV, but it was like the programme "Jackass". It was very funny. I kept losing him. There was lots of other stuff going on but can't remember what.

DAY 11

Nightmare 4.am
Lots of muddled dreams.

DAY 12

Muddled dreams. Felt I was being punished, like someone was doing this to me. Not punished for something I had done – they just wanted to hurt me.

DAY 23

Lots of dreams – water/swimming/oceans, rivers. Lots of activity.

Sycotic Co.

The keynote of Sycotic Co. is irritation

These are nervous, tense, stressed and easily upset people. They are often tearful and petulant when things go wrong. They are shy and withdrawn generally because they are emotionally vulnerable and very sensitive.

Sycotic co. are fussy people, everything must be just how they want it for them to be comfortable.

They are quick tempered if they think they are being criticised, and they are prone to think it. Resentment at this perceived slight leads to outburst of temper which can be violent.

They fear being neglected, being left alone. There is a fear of the dark especially when alone and of fierce animals especially dogs (there is a fear of a lack of civilization here, they want the world to be predictable). They have dreams of dead people and many scary nightmares.

There is a restlessness about their nature which leads them away from security but which makes them more anxious and fearful from its lack. Then they get exhausted by the strain of worrying. Leading them into ritual behaviour and stress reactions like nail biting.

They tend to fuss over things in the hope that attention to the detail will ensure success while avoiding the big picture. If you look at the ground in front of you then you might be able to ignore the Grand Canyon a few feet away. Anticipatory anxiety. They bite their nails from worry until it becomes a habit. They exaggerate their own importance to themselves as well as to others, and exaggerate the severity of their symptoms when reporting them.

Generalities

Restless. Nervy. They tend often to be plump

Overproduction of mucous. All systems easily disturbed.

Abundant perspiration at night yet feels chilly. Overgrowth of tissues.

Convulsions, epilepsy, meningitis and chorea; but not as frequently as Dys co.

Chilly and anaemic. Weariness and exhaustion. Anorexia.

Head

Persistent violent head pain like that of meningitis. Irritation of the meninges

Chronic headache which changes little and relieves rarely.

Headaches which are regular, weekly or monthly or with the menses

Throbbing headache < left side < noise, >heat >rest

Headaches from sinus problems.

Headaches which cause only a little pain but never completely go away.

Headache every weekend (Tub), which may persist for days. (pre-tubercular state)

Persistent headache in a child may be a feature of, or prodromal sign of, tubercular meningitis

Sick headache before during or after the menses

Irritability with special reference to synovial & mucus membrane

Premature grey hair

Alopecia

Sweaty head

Painful dry scaly spots on scalp

Premature greying of the hair

Face

Facial twitching and tics

Acne rosacea

Greasy skin.

Left sided facial neuralgias

Puffy in the morning especially under the eyes

Hair on face and upper lip.

Herpes around mouth.

Eczema of face from 4 months to 2 years of age

Swelling around eyes and of upper eyelids.

Eyes

Photophobia. Hemiopia. Tendency to blink a lot

Conjunctivitis. Tarsal cysts. Vitreous opacities

Pain in the eyeball

Ears
Deafness, otorrhea and excessive formation of wax
Cracks under or behind the ears
Itching in the meatus
Nose
Watery nasal cataarh, post nasal cataarh, blocked or obstructed thicker cataarh, dryness of the nose with crusts
Nasal polyps. Cracks at the angle of the nose.
Loss of sense of smell
Epistaxis
Pain in frontal and maxillary sinuses
Symptoms associated with, or aggravated by, hay fever.
Mouth and Taste
Cracks in the corner of mouth
Persistent herpes around mouth
Tongue sore/ulcerated/dry/warty. Ulcers tend to be deep.
Pins and needles of tongue
Excess salivation or tongue so dry that it sticks to the roof of the mouth
Sore tongue, feels scalded, can appear cracked.
Pins and needles in tongue
Lips dry and cracked
Loss of taste.
Throat
Overgrowth of tonsils
Cheesy tonsils Chokes easily
Recurrent tonsillitis with enlarged tonsils and adenoids
Throat feels raw, scorched and *dry*
Quinsy. (Peri tonsillar abscess)
Profuse mucous in throat in the morning
Swallowing difficult, chokes easily
Tough expectoration
External goitres.
Back and neck
Stiffness and pains, worse in the morning and in damp weather.
Sebaceous cysts.
Neuritis. Post herpetic neuralgia.
Pain in left scapula

Chest and heart

Pain in right lung. Intercostal neuralgia

Sharp pains in chest wall on inspiration.

Respiration and lungs

Wakes regularly through the night from cough. Wheeze, dyspnea and cough on waking

Coughs till sick. Bouts of croup at 2/4/6am

Cough comes in spasms and is affected by changes in the weather

Cough and wheezing <night, especially between 2 and 3am and at 4 and 6am. The child wakes with a croupy cough around these times.

Frequent bronchial colds. Cough with easy expectoration (or tough)

Head colds always go to chest

Asthma and bronchitis < damp and frosty weather and winter generally. > seaside

Pleurisy, Pleurodynia

Bronchial catarrh

Female

Uterine Polyps Ovarian cysts

Menorrhagia, metrorrhagia, dysmenorrhoea.

Offensive and profuse fishy leucorrhoea , alternatively profuse and bland.

Copious discharge yellowish, white or dark brown

Vulval pruritis, vaginitis

Pain in left ovary during menses

Tubal infections,

Genital warts and herpes.

Male

Genital warts and herpes

Pruritis

Balanitis

Impotence

Abdomen

Distention from flatulence.

Visceroptosis.

Stomach and digestion

Aversions; eggs, fat, milk, mild pudding, cream, salt, sugar, vegetables, tea, vinegar, cheese, meat, bread, potato and tomato. thought of breakfast makes him nauseous.

Desires; butter, fat, cheese, sweets, milk and salt

Finicky appetite, does not eat well. Tendency to anorexia/bulimia

Chronic irritation and catarrhal state of the whole alimentary tract (Med)

Burning pains. Nausea from eggs or cooking smells. Acid eructations, heartburn

Bilious attacks.

Pain and distension in the epigastrium

Pain right and left iliac fossa.

Kidneys and Urinary

Nephritis/pyelitis/cystitis

Burning and corrosive urine with very strong odour

Tendency to take urinary infection easily which spreads through the whole system.

Chronic cystitis.

Kidney pains

Nocturnal enuresis in children

Proteinuria, Nephritis, Cystitis, Pyelitis, Nephrosis; Renal colic

Frequency and urgency.

Rectum and stool

Acute and chronic gastro-enteritis

Watery stool after every meal.

Loose pale, frothy or crumbly stool may be offensive in odour and excoriating.

Urgent call to stool, when rising from bed

Mucous per rectum or with stool.

Distended feeling in the rectum, or splinter pains

Prolapse of rectum

Perianal warts. Condylomata around anus.

Copious flatulence

Urgency of stool may be brought on by excitement

Constipation or looseness. (Diarrhoea more common)

Sleep
Restless with many nightmares
Perspiration profuse on head and body 12-4am
Insomnia. Cannot get to sleep till 3am
Wakes 2-3am
Waking from cough or wheezing
Dreams of dead bodies.
Extremities
Neuralgia especially intercostals
Fibrositis of the shoulder. Neuritis in the arms.
Muscular rheumatism of the arms, shoulder, elbows and wrists.
Arthritis of wrists, fingers, pain>dry weather>hot water.
Fingers deformed by arthritis. Nodules on fingers.
Fingers go dead, numb. Prickly feeling in hands
Arthritis of metacarpo-phalangeal joints
Feet and legs painful at night
Rheumatism of knees. Bursitis
Ankles swollen and stiff. Feet swollen at night
Soles of feet painful when walking, they feel as if he was walking on loose cobble stones.
Big toe joint painful stiff and gouty.
Restless legs and feet in bed at night
Weakened nails.
General fibrositis, <damp<rest (Rhus Tox)
Skin
Sallow, greasy and a tendency to be indurated.
Vesicular rash related to Ant tart, Rhus Tox, Bacillinum and Thuja. (Think of this remedy in chicken pox)
Warty growths that may be large, flat and ragged and especially at the borders between mucosal and surface skin are typical for Sycotic-co.
Impetigo
Cracks on finger tips, cracks on heels
Nails brittle. Dermatitis of the palms; itchy<night<heat<excitement<flour<detergent
Eczema on the backs of the hands, pustules with heat and itching
Paronychia. Varicose eczema of ankles
Circinate eruptions on arms, thighs and shins
Chilblains <heat

Herpes face, neck and chest, groin
Varicellar eruption of limbs since immunisation
Intertrigo between breasts
Work related dermatitis

General Modalities

Everything < night
Chilly < damp < frost < humid weather. Change of weather.
> heat > seaside
<eggs, fat, onions and oranges

Related remedies

AntimonyTart	Kali Bich	Lycopodium	Natrum Mur
Natrum Sulph	Nitric Ac	Pulsatilla	Rhus Tox
Sepia	Thuja		

Afterword

It has been a labour of love, well at least a labour, completing my bowel nosodes work and I have now distilled all my bowel nosode cases into this Materia Medica and my other books. I would, however, be delighted to hear of cures, cases, problems raised and solved, and other bowel nosode information, and, in turn, I will be very happy to share any further knowledge that I gain.

Please feel free to contact me with any questions or information either on my email address saschanimmo@gmail.com or via facebook.

Anthony Bickley
Somerset
December 2017